MCQs on Clinical Pharmacology

MCQs on Clinical Pharmacology

D.R. Laurence MD FRCP
Professor of Pharmacology and Therapeutics,
Departments of Pharmacology and Clinical Pharmacology,
School of Medicine,
University College, London

P.N. Bennett MD FRCP
Consultant Physician,
Royal United Hospital, Bath
and Senior Lecturer in Clinical Pharmacology,
University of Bath

J.F. Stokes MD FRCP
Consulting Physician,
University College Hospital, London

CHURCHILL LIVINGSTONE
EDINBURGH LONDON MELBOURNE AND NEW YORK 1983

CHURCHILL LIVINGSTONE
Medical Division of Longman Group Limited

Distributed in the United States of America by Churchill
Livingstone Inc., 1560 Broadway, New York, N.Y.
10036, and by associated companies, branches and
representatives throughout the world.

© D.R. Laurence, P.N. Bennett & J.F. Stokes 1983

First published 1983

ISBN 0 443 02786 2

British Library Cataloguing in Publication Data
Laurence, D.R.
  MCQ's on clinical pharmacology.
  1. Pharmacology — Problems, exercises, etc.
  I. Title II. Bennett, P.N.
  III. Stokes, J.F.
  615.1'076   RM105

Library of Congress Cataloging in Publication Data
Laurence, D.R. (Desmond Roger)
  MCQs on Clinical pharmacology.
  'Questions are based on Clinical pharmacology (5th
edition) by D.R. Laurence and P.N. Bennett' — Pref.
  1. Pharmacology — Examinations, questions, etc. I.
Bennett, P.N. II. Stokes, J.F. (John Fisher) III. Laurence,
D.R. (Desmond Roger). Clinical pharmacology (5th ed.)
IV. Title. V. Title: M.C.Q.s on Clinical pharmacology.
[DNLM: 1. Pharmacology — Examination questions. QV
18 L379m]
RM300.L35   615'.7   82-4365
                               AACR2

Printed in Singapore by Huntsmen Offset Printing Pte Ltd

Preface

The *objective* of this book is to help students to acquire, and to know they have acquired, knowledge of clinical pharmacology which will be useful to them in practice and which is also sufficient for them to pass examinations.

The questions are based on *Clinical Pharmacology* (5th edition) by D.R. Laurence and P.N. Bennett (Churchill Livingstone) to which the reader may refer in order to check his answers and learn from his errors.

Although *the more experienced user* may attempt the questions as they stand with the object of testing the range of his knowledge, *the less experienced* may prefer to read a chapter of the book and, after an interval of some hours, try to answer the relevant questions. Wrong choices are best checked with the book as they are made, since the purpose is to learn, not merely to record a score.

In almost all cases the correct answer will be found either explicitly or by obvious implication in the text of the chapter being studied, but occasionally reference to another chapter will be needed. Drugs may feature in more than one chapter (e.g. β-adrenoceptor blocking agents) and, when a principle of pharmacokinetics or an adverse reaction is involved, chapters 8 and 9 will repay study. Use of the index is rarely needed, though educationally it is no bad thing to have to search beyond a single chapter for an answer.

Some of the questions are inevitably based on simple memory of facts, the building blocks of pharmacology and medicine. But, in producing these questions, we have tried not only to inform and remind, but also to illustrate principles. It will be found, therefore, that many apparently factual questions can be answered from knowledge of principles. (Principle = fundamental truth as a basis for reasoning: OED.) Questions are all of the familiar multiple True/False type in which any number of choices within each question may be correct.

1983

D.R.L.
P.N.B.
J.F.S.

Contents

1 Drug Therapy

1.1 In drug therapy, the following statements are correct:

A Efficacy and safety of a drug lie solely in its chemical nature

B Considerations of pharmacokinetics are important

C Drugs are the major causative factor in the decline of mortality from infectious diseases of the past 100 years

D The concept of benefit versus risk is central to proper practice

E Whenever a drug is given a risk is taken

1.2 Disease may be

A cured by a course of a drug

B suppressed or controlled, without cure, by a drug

C prevented by a drug

D worsened by a drug

E mimicked by a drug

1.3 Iatrogenic disease

A occurs as a result of self-medication

B occurs as a result of prescribed medication

C is a significant cause of admission to hospital

D may result from bad medical advice

E is caused by patient non-compliance with clear instructions

1.4   The following statements about drug therapy are correct:

A   In a patient with a self-limiting illness, it is still wiser to give a drug than to withold it, if in doubt

B   It is essentially irrational to use more than one drug for any single disease process

C   It is unlikely that more than three drugs will be taken reliably by most patients

D   Treatment should not be started until sufficient data have been collected to reach a rational decision

E   Therapeutic effects are more likely to be additive than adverse effects.

1.5   Risk

A   may be graded as unacceptable, acceptable or negligible

B   involved in using penicillin is such that it should only be used in life-endangering infections

C   if unnecessary, is avoided by most people in their daily life

D   is ignored by most people if it is less than 1:100 000

E   of death from a drug contraindicates its use

1.6   In evaluating adverse drug reactions as a source of disease it is useful to study their

A   nature

B   severity

C   incidence

D   avoidability

E   relationship to predisposing or causative factors in patients

1.7   In assessing the amount of disease that is caused by the practice of drug therapy the definition of an adverse drug reaction should include

A   any unwanted effect, however small

B   an effect that can be deemed actually harmful or seriously unpleasant

C   accidental or deliberate overdose
D   effects that warrant reduction of dose, withdrawal of the drug or foretell hazard from future administration
E   avoidable as well as unavoidable effects

1.8 The following statements are correct about data collecting methods:

A   Retrospective studies are expensive and time-consuming but provide reliable results
B   Prospective studies are easy and economical but are inherently unreliable
C   A case-control study involves comparing affected individuals with unaffected individuals who are comparable in other respects
D   A cohort study involves a substantial selected group of subjects monitored prospectively
E   Pre-marketing (licencing) drug therapeutic trials are insufficient to detect rare or late-developing adverse effects

1.9 In investigating the possibility of a drug-induced illness the finding that

A   a drug commonly induces an otherwise rare illlness is detectable only with the utmost difficulty
B   a drug rarely induces an otherwise common illness may go for ever undiscovered
C   a drug rarely induces an otherwise rare illness is likely to be detected early in pre-licencing clinical trials
D   a drug commonly induces an otherwise common illness is likely to be detected only in formal comparative studies
E   adverse reactions are relevant will be determined most reliably by clinical observation supported by case control and cohort studies

1.10 Adverse drug reactions

A cause 10% of consultations in general practice
B cause up to 3% of admissions to acute care hospital wards
C are particularly likely to occur in females over 60 years old
D are more likely to occur late rather than early in therapy
E are more likely to have a pharmacological rather than an immunological basis

1.11 Adverse drug reactions

A most commonly affect the cardiovascular and respiratory systems
B are not uncommon in patients taking digitalis and diuretics
C often affect the gastrointestinal tract and skin
D do not follow the use of a placebo
E will not occur if a drug has been correctly chosen even if it is incorrectly used

1.12 The following statements about liability for adverse effects of drugs are correct:

A Liability to compensate for injury of another person caused by negligence (fault) is usual in all legal systems
B If a patient suffers an adverse drug reaction, someone (the producer or prescriber, for instance) has been negligent
C It is easy to determine whether an adverse event or worsening of health is due to a drug
D Some adverse drug reactions could as readily be said to be due to a 'defect' in the patient as to a 'defect' in the drug
E Capacity to cause harm is inherent in even the most useful drugs

1.13 It is an accepted principle of 'product liability' that if the producer has given warning of a hazard associated with the use of the product then he is not liable to provide compensation if the injury warned against eventuates. If this is applied to drugs

A manufacturers would naturally insert into their Data Sheet every warning they could reasonably conjure up

B doctors would feel obliged to pass on every warning of adverse effects, however rare, to their patients

C patients would no longer leave the risk acceptance decision to the doctor

D doctors would be in a position to quantify risks with precision

E a patient suffering drug-induced injury could be counted on to agree that he had been warned and so was not entitled to compensation.

1.14 **Despite the manifest difficulties of providing special compensation for drug-caused injury, a scheme to meet public demand might be found socially and politically, acceptable if it incorporated the following concepts:**

A Liability for drugs under trial before being licenced for general use should fall on the producer

B Liability for recently licenced drugs should fall on a central fund provided jointly by the producer and the Government

C Liability for standard drugs should fall on a central fund

D Compensation in the case of standard drugs should only be for rare serious effects not ordinarily taken into account when prescribing the drug

E Prolonged legal argument may have to be accepted in cases of compensation for the effects of standard drugs

1.15 **The taking of drugs**

A is more likely to produce adverse reactions if therapy is prolonged

B is more likely to lead to withdrawal effect when treatment is stopped gradually rather than suddenly

C may put a patient at added risk from intercurrent disease

D may result in unfavourable interaction with items in the patient's diet

E both doctor-prescribed and self-prescribed has been increasing over the past ten years

1.16 When taking a patient's history it should be remembered that

A drugs can conceal disease
B drugs do not interfere with clinical chemistry tests
C response to drugs may give diagnostic clues
D withdrawal of drug therapy can cause disease
E drugs may leave residual effects after administration has ceased

1.17 The following statements about drug therapy are correct:

A The response in acute infections is much influenced by the interaction of the personalities of doctor and patient
B The response in anxiety or depression is primarily determined by the choice of drug and has little to do with the personal interaction of doctor, patient and social environment
C Response to a drug can be significantly affected by the initial level of activity of the target organ or system
D It is of no consequence what sort of medicine the patient thinks he has been given, all that matters is what he has in fact been given
E Knowledge of *why* a patient gets better is of purely academic interest

1.18 A placebo effect

A may follow treatment of all kinds
B only occurs in mentally ill patients
C is likely to recur regularly in a placebo reactor
D can be expected in about 35% of patients
E following a tonic usually has a distinct pharmacological basis

1.19 Placebo reactors tend to be

A introverted
B unsociable
C acquiescent

D lacking in self-confidence
E neurotic

1.20 **Factors established as being associated with patient non-compliance include**

A lack of understanding of instructions
B psychiatric illness
C prescription of more than three drugs
D inconvenient clinics
E family instability

1.21 **Medicines in the home**

A in most cases are non-prescribed
B are found in about one house in ten
C are usually kept in a locked cupboard or drawer, inaccessible to children
D are most commonly kept in the bathroom
E should be confined to those suitable for short-term relief of symptoms, such as analgesics, except where a medicine is in use according to medical direction.

2 Clinical Pharmacology

2.1 **Clinical pharmacology, the scientific study of drugs in man**

A   is a discipline called into existence by need
B   comprises pharmacodynamics, pharmacokientics, formal therapeutic trials and surveillance studies
C   is so complex that it can only be conducted by specialist clinical pharmacologists
D   raises problems that require experiments in animals for elucidation
E   is fundamentally different from basic pharmacological science conducted on non-human animals or tissues

3 How Drugs Act

3.1 **The following statements about how drugs act are correct:**

A Living creatures, plants and animals, often produce toxic substances the effect of which is confined to their own genus

B The heart of modern pharmacology is selective action between tissues

C An inhibitor of enzyme-mediated synthesis is a substance that fits one active site of an enzyme but which is sufficiently unlike the usual substrate to fail to react with the substrate molecule fitted into the adjacent active site

D An inhibitor of enzyme-mediated degradation is a substance that fits an active site of an enzyme so that its natural substrate remains intact

E When a molecule offered to an enzyme is so similar to its normal substrate that it can be used in synthetic reaction, the product may be biologically active, e.g. as a false transmitter

3.2 **The following statements about how drugs act are correct:**

A Drugs may alter the flow of ions across cell membranes

B Substances specially needed by cells may be subject to special active chemical pumping mechanisms

C Cells are provided with special macromolecular sites the conformation of which fits specific chemicals and which activate biological processes within the cell. These are called receptors

D There is only one type of receptor for each chemical transmitter or drug

E As concentration rises drugs become less selective and unwanted effects increasingly appear

4 Discovery and Development of New Drugs

4.1 In discovering and developing new drugs

A the most likely way of discovering a really novel drug is to precisely define natural biochemical mechanisms and to synthesise substances that annul or mimic them

B modification of structures of existing drugs is likely to provide modest improvements such as greater ease of use

C knowledge of mode of action of a drug is not particularly useful for predicting effects in man from studies in animals

D induction of experimental diseases in animals (such as hypertension or arthritis) provides an ideal test system for studies predictive for man

E knowledge of kinetics of a drug in a test species allows toxicology tests to be designed with maximum relevance to use of the drug in man

4.2 In the development of new drugs

A differences in drug response between species, including man, are more commonly pharmacodynamic than pharmacokinetic

B a crude measure of safety of a drug may be obtained by dividing the ED_{50} by the LD_{50}

C toxicity tests in animals are generally confined to 6 months duration (except for oncogenicity) even though the drugs may be used in man for years

D testing of all new drugs on pregnant animals has been mandatory since the thalidomide disaster

E national registers of birth defects, competently kept, plus accurate records of drug consumption should ensure that no serious drug-induced defect in the fetus will be overlooked

4.3 **The following statements about mutagenesis and oncogenesis are correct:**

A Testing in animals for oncogenicity and mutagenicity should be mandatory for all new drugs, even those that are intended for short-term use

B If a drug is mutagenic this effect will be detectable early during its administration

C Mutagens may also be carcinogens

D Drug-induced cancer may occur many years after the patient has stopped using the drug

E Anti-cancer drugs are also carcinogenic

4.4 **The following statements about special toxicology (reproduction, mutagenesis, carcinogenesis) are correct:**

A If a drug is teratogenic in an animal species it may not be used in women of reproductive age

B A positive laboratory mutagenicity test should bar the use of a substance in humans

C If the first generation offspring of a male human are normal then a mutagenic effect on his reproductive cells has not occurred

D Some drugs that are carcinogenic are in use in routine therapy

E If a drug is under suspicion for carcinogenicity (or mutagenicity or teratogenicity) a case control study is likely to be helpful

4.5 **The following statements about new drugs are correct:**

A The scientific basis of new drug development is to predict from experiments in animals what their effects in man will be

B Human diseases are usually easily mimicked in laboratory animals

C Toxicity testing in animals should be undertaken regardless of expense even if there is doubt about the relevance of the results to man

D It is possible to spend too much time in animal studies before a drug is tested in man

E All drug actions can be demonstrated in healthy volunteers

4.6   Rational introduction of a potential new drug comprises

A   pharmacological study on healthy subjects or patients
B   wider use on patients to detect potential therapeutic utility
C   formal controlled trials
D   monitoring for adverse reactions (and efficacy) after release for general prescribing
E   the submission of all research studies in man to an ethics review committee

5 Evaluation of Drug Therapy

5.1 **The following statements about the evaluation of drugs are correct:**

A If a drug produces a desired pharmacological action then it will be useful in therapeutics

B No drug should be licenced for general prescription until a true therapeutic effect has been shown, even if this takes years

C Since formal therapeutic trials cannot be conducted on sufficient numbers and kinds of patients to reveal all the effects of drugs it is essential to develop (postmarketing) surveillance techniques

D Formal therapeutic trials generally show the best that a drug can do in carefully selected patients. Surveillance studies provide knowledge of the drug under the conditions of ordinary medical practice

E It is important to include special classes of patient eg renal failure, pregnancy in the therapeutic trials conducted before licencing for general use (marketing)

5.2 **In the clinical evaluation of therapy the following statements are correct:**

A Physicians who follow their judgement aided only by personal experience and intuition are not engaging in experiments

B A scientific experimental approach to therapeutics is inherently less ethical than practice guided by clinical experience and impression

C General impressions are never to be trusted

D Clinical impressions are always wrong

E If a patient gets better after treatment it is reasonable to conclude that the recovery is due to the treatment

5.3   Therapeutic trials are designed to show as far as is practicable

A   whether a treatment is of value
B   how great is its value
C   in what type of patients it is of value
D   what is the best method of applying the treatment
E   what are the principal disadvantages or dangers of a treatment

5.4   Features of the classic randomized controlled therapeutic trial include

A   precisely framed question to be answered
B   equivalent groups of patients
C   groups formed by allocating alternate patients to each treatment under investigation
D   treatments carried out concurrently
E   double-blind technique where evaluation depends on strictly objective measurements

5.5   Placebo or dummy medication

A   provides a control device by which true pharmacodynamic effects of therapy are distinguised from the general psychological effects of medication
B   provides a device to avoid false negative conclusions
C   can be unethical
D   is always scientifically necessary in a trial of drug therapy
E   is sometimes used in patients who also receive a pharmacologically active treatment

5.6   In a therapeutic trial

A   different treatments must never be given to the same patient
B   the order in which treatments are given may influence the results

C the theoretical basis of the design is to test the hypothesis that there is no difference between the treatments under test

D there is a risk of finding a difference where there is in reality no difference

E there is no risk of finding no difference where there is in reality a difference

5.7   A statistical significance test

A is a device concerned with probabilities rather than with certainties

B when positive, tells us that a difference is clinically important

D applies to Type I errors

D cannot be of use in cross-over studies

E showing P = 0.05 means that if the experiment were repeated 100 times, there being in reality no difference between the treatments, then a difference as great as that observed would occur 5 times as a result of chance

5.8   A statistician

A can salvage a poorly designed experiment after it has been completed

B cannot tell the clinician how many patients he will need in a therapeutic trial to get a clinically important result unless the clinician can be explicit on the differences he expects and the risk he is prepared to accept of getting a misleading result

C can extract reliable information from old case records of treatment

D prefers sequential analysis to reliably detect small differences

E is likely to advise that a simple significance test conducted at regular intervals, the trial ceasing as soon as a positive result is obtained, is the best way of deciding when to stop a trial

5.9 **The following statements about therapeutic trials are correct:**

A Knowledge of the results of a therapeutic trial conducted in groups of patients does not help the physician faced with an individual patient

B A clinician who is personally convinced that treatment A is better than treatment B cannot ethically engage in a scientific study on the subject

C Once a therapeutic trial has given a positive result it becomes unethical to do another similar trial

D To conduct a scientific study in which the patient's treatment is chosen by random allocation is inherently unethical

E A good guide to conduct is that no patient participating in a therapeutic trial should be worse off than he might otherwise have been in the hands of a competent doctor

6 Drug Regulation or Control

6.1   The following statements about official drug regulation are correct:

A   Modern comprehensive official drug regulation began in the USA (1938) after an accident involving sulphanilamide and diethylene glycol

B   The company marketing the mixture tested it for fragrance and flavour but not for safety

C   The lack of testing for safety did not infringe the then law

D   The rest of the world only accepted the need for comprehensive control following the thalidomide disaster (1961)

E   No new drug should be licenced for general prescribing (marketed) until it has been proved safe

6.2   Official drug regulation or control is concerned with

A   quality of the manufactured drug and formulation

B   safety of the drug

C   efficacy of the drug

D   supply to the medical profession and the public

E   compiling a register of accepted medicinal products

6.3   A modern drug regulatory authority requires evidence of

A   studies on animals

B   chemical and pharmaceutical quality

C   pharmacological studies in man

D   formal therapeutic trials

E   post licencing (marketing) surveillance

6.4 **The following statements about thalidomide are correct:**

A New drugs were routinely tested on pregnant animals before the thalidomide disaster

B Thalidomide caused major anatomical abnormalities in fetuses

C Testing of new drugs for effects on reproduction may be confined to the period of organogenesis without losing capacity to predict risks to the fetus

D Thalidomide was recognised as harmful to fetuses as early as it was because it caused a very severe effect that was ordinarily seen extremely rarely

E When thalidomide was first suspected a case control study was quickly done

7 Classification of Drugs, Names of Drugs

7.1 The following statements are correct:

A   Classification is a fundamental requirement of a science
B   If classification is fundamental then it follows that nomenclature also is
C   A drug or medicine generally has three names
D   Proprietary names apply rather to formulations than to pure substances
E   There is a single classification of drugs that suits all interested parties

7.2 Drugs are generally classified by their

A   therapeutic use
B   adverse effects
C   mode of action
D   chemical structure
E   proprietary names

7.3 The following statements about nomenclature of drugs are correct:

A   Proprietary names are chosen to emphasise the difference between similar drugs
B   Official (non-proprietary) names are chosen to emphasise the similarity between related drugs
C   The full chemical name is best for prescribing purposes
D   There is never a medically important reason for using a proprietary name in prescribing
E   The majority of mixtures of drugs do not have non-proprietary names

8 General Pharmacology

8.1 Drugs act by

A combining with specific receptors
B inhibiting enzymes
C direct chemical reaction
D interfering with metabolic processes
E their physico-chemical (e.g. osmotic) properties

8.2 Competitive antagonism

A can be reversed by increasing the amount of agonist present
B can be said to be present when the log-dose-response curve to agonist alone is not parallel to the curve obtained when an antagonist is present
C generally involves substances that are comparatively inactive themselves
D never occurs with enzymes
E cannot easily be distinguished from physiological antagonism

8.3 Selectivity of drug action

A is a disadvantage in anticancer chemotherapy
B is undesirable because it limits the number of conditions for which a drug may be used
C is a concept which partly owes its origins to weedkillers
D is the underlying principle of Paul Ehrlich's 'magic bullet'
E is exhibited by histamine H_2-receptor antagonists

8.4   The plasma t½ of a drug is

A   a fundamental concept in pharmacokinetics

B   the time in which the concentration of drug in plasma declines by one half

C   the same as its biological t½

D   usually lengthened if biologically active metabolites are formed

E   likely to be altered in hepatic disease if the liver is the normal route of elimination

8.5   The following statements about drug t½ are correct:

A   A drug which is reabsorbed by the renal tubules is likely to have a longer t½ than one which is not reabsorbed by the renal tubules

B   A drug which has a low free plasma concentration because of extensive binding to plasma protein and to tissues is likely to have a short t½

C   Extent of drug distribution e.g. into total body water or into extracellular fluid, is unlikely to affect t½

D   A drug which is actively secreted by the renal tubules is likely to have a longer t½ than one which is not actively secreted

E   The plasma t½ of a 'hit and run' drug is very much shorter than its duration of action

8.6   First order processes

A   only apply to enzyme-mediated reactions

B   are characterised by high rates of reaction when the concentrations of reacting substances are high and *vice versa*

C   can properly be described in terms of t½

D   give rise to dose dependent kinetics

E   are involved in the metabolism of alcohol only at high plasma concentrations

8.7 **When the kinetics of a drug are described by zero order processes**

A elimination rate is independent of dose
B t½ is constant despite rising drug concentration
C the elimination processes have become saturated
D uniform increases in dose may result in disproportionate increases in plasma concentration
E the Law of Mass Action applies

8.8 **The following statements about phenytoin are correct:**

A Kinetics change from first order to zero order at doses below or within the therapeutic range
B When kinetics are first order, increments in dose result in disproportionate rise in plasma concentration
C When kinetics become zero order measurement of plasma concentration becomes unnecessary
D Alteration in the diluent in the capsule in which it is prescribed can affect absorption
E Its membrane stabilising properties are valuable in the control of cardiac dysrhythmias

8.9 **Drug clearance by the body**

A only refers to elimination by the kidney
B refers to the volume of blood cleared of drug in unit time
C cannot exceed glomerular filtration rate
D may be influenced by renal tubular secretion
E is in principle the same as creatinine clearance

8.10 **For a drug to be transferred across cell membranes**

A by diffusion, active energy-requiring processes are required
B by active transport, it is essential that the drug be lipid soluble and unionized
C by filtration, the drug passes through pores in the membrane

D lipid solubility is an advantage
E it must first be metabolized

8.11 The following statements about drug ionization are correct:

A If a drug is 50% ionized and 50% unionized, the pH of its environment is equal to its pKa
B Every drug must have its own pKa because all drugs contain readily ionizable chemical groups
C The extent to which a chemical group tends to ionize can be expressed as the dissociation constant or Ka
D The pKa is the negative logarithm of the Ka
E Aspirin (pKa 3.5) is 91% unionized at pH 2.5

8.12 The following statements are correct:

A Acid groups become less ionized in an acid medium
B Unionized drug is lipid insoluble and non-diffusible
C Two drugs which have ionizable groups of the same pKa will automatically have the same lipid solubility
D pKa varies with environmental pH
E Many drugs are weak electrolytes

8.13 Aspirin (pKa 3.5)

A will be unionized in the stomach (pH 1.5)
B will be unionized in the small intestine (pH 6.8–7.6)
C is more rapidly eliminated by the kidney if a high urine pH is maintained
D is mainly absorbed from the small intestine
E remains predominantly in extracellular fluid because this is slightly more alkaline than the intracellular environment

8.14 Administration of certain drugs by mouth may be less effective than by parenteral administration

A because of destruction of drug within the gut
B because of rapid metabolism of drug in the gut wall or liver before reaching the systemic circulation
C because of active absorption of drug by the small intestine.
D because food may interfere with drug absorption
E because anticholinergics may delay absorption

8.15 Rectal administration of drugs

A is more effective because absorption into the portal system and first pass elimination in the liver are avoided
B usually necessitates smaller doses than oral administration to achieve the same effect
C may be useful in migraine
D may cause proctitis
E is useful with drugs that irritate the stomach

8.16 Because blood flow is an important determinant of drug distribution

A adverse effects may occur after intravenous injection as the brain and heart are high blood flow organs
B rate of intravenous injection is unimportant
C muscular exercise may increase drug mobilisation after i.m. injection and cause adverse effects
D the intravenous route is preferred to the intramuscular route in peripheral circulatory failure
E subcutaneous injection is preferable to intramuscular injection for rapid onset of effect

8.17 Drug distribution may be influenced by

A body fluid pH
B regional blood flow
C plasma protein binding

D lipid solubility.

E binding in tissues other than blood

8.18 **The following statements about drug distribution are correct:**

A Volatile anaesthetics, being lipid soluble, tend to remain in the extracellular space

B Gentamicin, which is water soluble, passes readily into the cerebrospinal fluid

C Specialised transport mechanisms influence the distribution of iodine

D DDT and thiopentone do not distribute to fat

E Phenothiazine drugs distribute differentially to tissues

8.19 **The apparent volume of distribution**

A of a drug is the fluid volume which would contain the known dose of administered drug if the measured plasma concentration were uniform throughout all the tissues of the body

B of a drug refers to a specific anatomical space

C of digoxin is greater than body volume which indicates that this drug is selectively concentrated in tissues

D of aspirin is 12 litres in a 70 kg individual which suggests that the drug remains in extracellular fluid

E of antipyrine (phenazone) is approximately equal to total body water

8.20 **On the basis of apparent volume of distribution (Vd), haemodialysis would be effective in removing drug from subjects overdosed with**

A propranolol (Vd 250 litres/70 kg individual)

B chlorpromazine (Vd 1400 litres/70 kg individual)

C aspirin (Vd 12 litres/70 kg individual)

D digoxin (Vd 500 litres/70 kg individual)

E amitriptyline (Vd 2000 litres/70 kg individual)

8.21 Transfer of drug from blood to cerebrospinal fluid

A   is selective because continuous intercellular junctions ensure that drug must pass through cells to reach the brain

B   is largely limited to water-soluble drugs

C   for gentamicin and penicillin is greater if meninges are inflamed

D   may involve active transport mechanisms

E   in the case of anti-tuberculosis agents is so poor that intrathecal administration is mandatory in all cases of tuberculous meningitis

8.22 Drug bound to plasma protein

A   is pharmacologically inactive

B   can only be removed by metabolism of the binding protein

C   is not available for metabolism until it has dissociated from the protein

D   in the case of warfarin is 10%

E   in the case of phenylbutazone is 98%

8.23 Extent of drug binding to plasma proteins

A   may be reduced in renal disease because the capacity of individual albumin molecules to bind drug is reduced

B   is relatively unaffected by hypoalbuminaemia in the cases of digoxin and frusemide

C   is indicated by measuring total drug concentration in plasma

D   may limit the effectiveness of diazoxide given i.v.

E   is greatly influenced by genetic factors

8.24 Displacement of a drug from its protein binding site

A   can be assumed if two highly protein-bound drugs are administered together

B   may be caused by natural blood constituents such as bilirubin and fatty acids

C is more likely to cause a clinically important drug interaction if the concentration of the displaced drug requires to be precisely controlled

D is unlikely to lead to adverse effects in the case of warfarin

E in the case of tolbutamide may be sufficient to cause hypoglycaemia

8.25 Drug metabolizing enzymes

A in general act to produce molecules having lessened solubility in water

B were probably successful evolutionary mechanisms since they permit the body to dispose of lipid soluble substances ingested in foods

C are individually specific for particular drugs

D are generally absent from fish which can lose lipid-soluble substances through the gills

E are present in the intestinal mucosa

8.26 Drug metabolism

A can take place in lung

B invariably results in loss of pharmacological activity

C proceeds at the same rates in twins whether they are monovular or binovular

D rates for some antidepressants may vary ten-fold or more between individuals

E in the liver greatly limits the access of some drugs to the systemic circulation after oral administration

8.27 Enzyme induction

A occurs in both hepatic and extrahepatic tissues

B develops within days of administration of an inducing agent

C is usually brought about by lipid insoluble substances with short half-life

D enables the body to adapt to varying exposure to foreign compounds

E can be a cause of loss of anticoagulant control

8.28 Enzyme induction

A with anticonvulsants may cause osteomalacia
B contributes to tolerance to the effects of ethanol
C can cause failure of the contraceptive pill
D may occur as a result of smoking
E can affect plasma bilirubin concentration

8.29 The following statements about drugs in breast milk are correct:

A Drug may partition into breast milk because the pH of milk differs from that of blood
B Diazepam taken by a mother may pass into her milk in amounts sufficient to affect the baby
C Temazepam ingested breast milk is unlikely to cause adverse effects in the baby because its metabolites are inactive
D Replacement hormones taken by a mother may pass into her milk in amounts sufficient to affect the baby adversely
E A mother who is taking chloramphenicol should not breast-feed her infant

8.30 Plasma concentration

A of phenytoin in a group of individuals can be expected to be very similar if each receives a standard 300 mg oral dose
B measurement is useful to monitor diuretic therapy
C of most drugs correlates better with clinical effect than does dose
D measurements may explain failure of therapeutic effect when conventional doses of drug are administered
E measurements are of no value when drug elimination mechanisms are impaired

8.31 **Drug plasma concentration is likely to be useless or misleading**

A   in the case of digoxin if the blood sample is taken 0-4 hours after dosing

B   in the case of drugs which bind irreversibly to target tissue, e.g. monoamine oxidase

C   if the assay technique measures inactive metabolites.

D   if the assay technique fails to measure active metabolites

E   in the case of lithium because it has a long t½

8.32 **The kidney is vulnerable to toxic injury**

A   because drug concentration in urine is generally much higher than that in blood

B   because relatively high drug concentration is achieved in the renal medulla by a counter-current mechanism.

C   because drug induced immune complexes are filtered by the kidney

D   from gold salts

E   from the use of uricosuric drugs

8.33 **The following drugs are eliminated unchanged by the kidney:**

A   Lignocaine

B   Lithium

C   Gentamicin

D   Chlorpromazine

E   Levodopa

8.34 **The fact that the following drugs are eliminated almost exclusively by non-renal mechanisms is important in prescribing for patients with renal failure:**

A   Propranolol

B   Cephalexin

C   Doxycycline

D   Phenytoin

E   Methotrexate

8.35 When renal function is impaired

A   for drugs highly dependent on the kidney for elimination, creatinine clearance can be used as a guide to change in half-life

B   raised plasma creatinine is an indication to reduce the dose of drugs that are eliminated by the kidney

C   reduced doses based on plasma creatinine value will suffice for short courses of drugs

D   if a drug is given at a constant rate, it will take less than the normal four half-lives to reach 93.75% of ultimate steady state

E   tetracycline is best avoided

8.36 In patients with renal disease

A   a reduced dose of digoxin is usually required

B   diuretics acting principally on the distal renal tubule are the most effective

C   antacids should be checked for sodium and potassium content

D   allopurinol is not effective in the prophylaxis of gout

E   propranolol is contraindicated for the control of hypertension

8.37 The following statements about drugs and the liver are correct:

A   Jaundice due to C-17 substituted testosterone derivatives is dose-related

B   Androgens that are active only by injection do not cause jaundice

C   Jaundice due to a hydrazine derivative such as isoniazid may occur up to three weeks after stopping the drug

D   Cholestatic injury due to phenothiazines usually resolves

E   Liver cell injury due to paracetamol is part of generalised drug allergy

8.38 In patients with liver disease

A adverse response to centrally acting drugs is due to abnormality of brain cells as much as or more than to failure of the liver to metabolize drugs

B morphine is a satisfactory analgesic

C a benzodiazepine with short t½ and inactive metabolites should be used if sedation is essential

D theophylline usually has a normal t½

E diuretic therapy presents no greater hazard than in patients without liver disease

8.39 The following statements about steady state or plateau drug concentration are correct:

A 75% of ultimate steady state is reached in two drug t½s

B If the dose is doubled the time to reach steady state is doubled

C The time to reach steady state is a function of t½ and dose

D If a drug is given until steady state plasma concentration has been attained and the dose is then doubled, the new steady state level will be double the original level

E If a drug is given until steady state plasma concentration has been attained and the dose is then altered, a new steady state will be reached in about four t½s

8.40 A loading or priming dose

A is smaller than the maintenance dose

B is equal to the amount of drug which is eliminated in a dose interval

C is unnecessary for benzylpenicillin (t½ 30 minutes)

D is necessary if a rapid onset of action of digoxin (t½ 36-48 hours) is required

E is given with the objective of achieving quickly the desired drug concentration in the body

8.41 Fixed-dose drug combinations for systemic use

A are advantageous when drugs have a synergistic effect
B are best used for drugs with narrow dose-range
C improve compliance with therapy
D of iron, folic acid and cyanocobalamin are hazardous
E including adrenocortical steroids should not be used

8.42 Biological availability

A is indicated by the area under the plasma concentration-time curve
B of a drug which is injected intravenously must be less than 100%
C may be reduced by destruction of drug in the gut
D may be reduced by metabolism of drug in the liver
E is unlikely to be affected by particle size of the pharmaceutical formulation

8.43 The following statements are correct:

A Drug A is more potent than drug B if drug A can achieve a greater maximum effect than drug B
B Drug A is more efficacious than drug B if weight for weight drug A has a greater effect than drug B
C Differences in potency are often without clinical importance
D Bumetanide 1 mg achieves about the same diuretic effect as frusemide 40 mg — the drugs therefore have approximately equal potency
E Frusemide has greater therapeutic efficacy than thiazide diuretics because it can produce a diuresis where a thiazide fails

8.44 Biological assay

A is a process by which the activity of a substance, identified or unidentified, is measured on living material
B is generally preferable to chemical or physical methods of assay if both are available

C   ought not to be employed if the dose response curves of reference and test substances are not parallel
D   is a term which could be applied to clinical trials
E   is usually too insensitive to be of practical value

8.45   Genetically determined variation in drug response between individuals

A   shows a continuous distribution if multifactorial
B   shows a discontinuous distribution if monofactorial
C   may explain phenytoin toxicity at normal doses
D   may explain failure of rat poison to kill some rats
E   is normally greater for identical than for non-identical twins

8.46   Interaction between drugs

A   with steep dose response curves is unlikely to be harmful
B   with small therapeutic ratios is unlikely to be harmful
C   is described as summation if the effects of two drugs with the same action are additive
D   is described as potentiation if the action of one drug increases the effect of another
E   may lead to valuable therapeutic effects

8.47   Addition of drugs to intravenous fluids

A   causes visible change in the solution if interaction is occurring
B   is safe in the case of heparin with penicillin
C   is safe if the mixture is kept for several days before use
D   is acceptable for blood, aminoacid solutions and fat emulsions
E   may be rendered unsafe by the acidity of dextrose or sodium solutions

8.48 Interactions of drugs in the gut may occur due to

A changes in pH
B changes in motility
C direct chemical reaction
D alteration of gut flora
E alteration of mucosal absorptive mechanisms

8.49 Drug interaction between

A naloxone and morphine occurs principally at plasma protein binding sites
B monoamine oxidase inhibitors and levodopa may lead to hypotension
C tricyclic antidepressants and antihypertensives may result in loss of antihypertensive effect
D phenylbutazone and warfarin may lead to risk of bleeding
E neomycin and curare may cause increased neuromuscular blockade

8.50 The following statements about clinically significant interactions resulting from enzyme inhibition by drugs are correct:

A Drugs classed as monoamine oxidase inhibitors alter clinical responses to sympathomimetics alone
B Metronidazole and sulphonylureas alter clinical effects of alcohol
C Allopurinol reduces azathioprine metabolism
D Chloramphenicol reduces warfarin metabolism
E Phenylbutazone reduces tolbutamide metabolism

8.51 Alteration of urine pH

A with probenecid reduces elimination of penicillin and can be therapeutically useful
B can significantly affect the elimination of drugs which do not possess inonizable chemical groups.
C is valuable in overdose with aspirin

D with alkali is useful in detecting amphetamine addicts since it increases urinary elimination of the drug
E is of major importance in the management of overdose with pethidine

8.52 Metabolism of

A codeine leads to the formation of morphine
B benorylate terminates its analgesic effect
C talampicillin terminates its antibacterial effect
D phenylbutazone produces an active metabolite
E cyclophosphamide is essential for its biological effect

8.53 Interactions between drugs

A only take place within the body
B can only occur when drugs have the same site of action
C are invariably harmful
D may be antagonistic
E may be synergistic

9 Unwanted Effects of Drugs, Adverse Reactions

9.1 **The following statements about unwanted effects of drugs (adverse reactions) are correct:**

A There is a fundamental biological distinction between therapeutic and adverse effects of drugs

B Some adverse effects are due to normal predictable pharmacological effects of drugs and may occur in all patients taking the drug

C Some adverse effects are due to abnormalities in the patient and will only occur in some patients taking the drug

D The terms intolerant and tolerant refer to individuals at either extreme of the normal distribution curve

E Idiosyncrasy means allergy

9.2 **Factors which may influence the incidence of adverse reactions to drugs include:**

A Age
B Sex
C Genetic makeup
D Disease
E Tendency to allergy

9.3 **Adverse drug reactions are influenced by**

A inherent properties of the drug
B the choice of drug in a particular patient
C the way the drug is used
D the technique of manufacture of the pure drug
E other drugs the patient is taking

9.4 The following statements about adverse drug reactions are correct:

A Pharmacokinetic mechanisms are unimportant in causation
B Young children can be regarded as 'small adults' as far as liability to adverse drug reactions is concerned
C The first month of life is a period of special risk
D Old age is a period of special risk
E Older children metabolize some drugs more rapidly than do adults.

9.5 The elderly show an increased response to standard drug dosage and an increased incidence of adverse drug reactions because they have

A increased lean body mass
B reduced renal and hepatic function
C reduced blood flow to vital organs
D better nutrition
E less efficient homeostatic mechanisms

9.6 Patients having the following conditions tend to show a greater than normal response to many drugs:

A Hypoalbuminaemia
B Congestive cardiac failure
C Hepatic cirrhosis
D Hyperthyroidism
E Hypothyroidism

9.7 Hepatic porphyrias are due to hereditary single enzyme defects. Great attention to prescribing is necessary if serious drug-induced illness is to be avoided. An attack of porphyria may be precipitated by

A aspirin
B morphine
C barbiturates
D chlorpromazine
E some 'home remedies' e.g. mouthwash

9.8 **The following statements are correct:**

A   A hypnotic is better than an analgesic for a patient sleepless due to pain

B   A patient having rheumatic fever with heart failure should be treated with sodium salicylate

C   In peripheral circulatory failure from any cause drugs should not be injected subcutaneously

D   Hypopituatry patients are unusually tolerant of many drugs

E   In Hodgkin's lymphoma alcohol taken in social doses is liable to induce pain

9.9 **A healthy person whose work is in a surgical operating theatre and who lives an active easy-going social life is liable to absorb medically significant amounts of the following:**

A   Halothane
B   Penicillin
C   Dicophane (DDT)
D   Alcohol
E   Tobacco

9.10 **The following statements about drug allergy are correct:**

A   All drugs are antigens

B   If antibodies to a drug are present in a patient then he will suffer from an adverse reaction if he receives the drug again

C   Drugs or drug metabolites combine with a body protein to form an antigen

D   20% of adverse drug reactions have an immunological basis

E   The chief target organs of drug allergy are skin, respiratory tract, gastrointestinal tract, blood, blood vessels

9.11 **Where a drug causes an allergic (immunological) illness**

A it is safe to change to another member of the same chemical class

B there is no linear relation of dose to effect

C safe desensitization is impossible

D re-exposure to a small dose is enough to cause illness

E this illness mimics the principal pharmacological actions of the drug

9.12 **Important manifestations of drug allergy include**

A thrombocytopenia

B granulocytopenia/agranulocytosis

C leukaemia

D aplastic anaemia

E haemolysis

9.13 **Important manifestations of drug allergy include**

A serum sickness syndrome

B asthma

C fever

D hay fever

E collagen disease(s)

9.14 **Important manifestations of drug allergy include**

A peptic ulcer

B eczematous rash

C anaphylactic shock

D urticaria

E hepatitis/cholestasis

9.15 In drug allergy

A diagnosis rests primarily on laboratory tests

B after recovery from a reaction, rechallenge with the suspected drug is both essential and safe

C skin tests give reliable diagnostic information for contact dermatitis only

D detection of drug-specific circulating antibodies is diagnostically conclusive that a suspected reaction was indeed allergic

E once allergy has occurred it is permanent

9.16 Anaphylactic shock is an immunological condition in which

A interaction of antigen with antibody causes cell damage with release of biologically active substances

B histamine is an important cause of the shock

C the blood pressure falls dramatically

D the bronchi dilate dramatically

E the emergency treatment is adrenaline given intramuscularly followed by a histamine H_1-receptor antagonist followed by an adrenocortical steroid

9.17 Prevention of allergic reactions to drugs is assisted by

A ensuring patients are clearly informed that they have an allergy

B paying attention to what patients tell you

C doing weekly blood counts on patients taking any drug known to produce blood disorders

D always taking a drug history from all patients

E desensitizing (hyposensitizing) all patients suspected of penicillin allergy

9.18 In early pregnancy

A drugs may damage the embryo or fetus by direct action on it or indirectly by altering the mother's physiology

B the placenta readily allows water-soluble drugs to pass from mother to fetus

C once a drug enters the fetus it tends to persist longer than in the mother

D therapeutic effects on the fetus are sometimes achieved by giving drugs to the mother

E teratogens are likely to have their most devastating effects

9.19 In late pregnancy

A gross anatomical defects in the fetus are likely to result from drugs

B non-steroidal anti-inflammatory drugs can delay the onset of labour

C a vasoconstrictor drug given to the mother can cause fetal distress

D opiates given to the mother do not affect the fetus

E benzodiazepines given to the mother do not affect the fetus

9.20 The following statements about the relationship between drugs and fetal abnormalities are correct:

A If a drug is suspected of causing fetal abnormality a case control study will be useful

B When prescribing, it is as important to consider whether a woman may become pregnant as whether she is already pregnant

C Some drugs in common use may be low grade teratogens

D If a baby is born with an anatomical abnormality it should be possible to attribute it to a drug

E Fetal abnormality may be due to the disease for which the drug was prescribed

9.21 Substances strongly suspected or known to be capable of harming the fetus when consumed by a pregnant woman include

A penicillin

B sex hormones

C antiepileptics

D anticoagulants

E alcohol

10 Chemotherapy and Chemotherapeutic Agents

10.1 The following drugs are primarily bactericidal:

A Sulphonamides
B Tetracyclines
C Aminoglycosides
D Chloramphenicol
E Rifampicin

10.2 The following statements about the mechanism of antimicrobial drug action are correct:

A Penicillin interferes with the peptidoglycan layer of the cell so that it absorbs water and bursts
B Amphotericin interferes with the cytoplasmic membrane of fungi
C Sulphonamides interfere with the build-up of peptide chains on ribosomes
D Tetracyclines prevent bacteria from synthesising folic acid
E Rifampicin interferes with bacterial nucleic acid metabolism

10.3 The choice of antimicrobial drugs

A may follow automatically from the clinical diagnosis if the causative organism is always the same and is always sensitive to the same drug
B should always be delayed until a positive identification of the infecting organism has been made
C should be based exclusively on *in vitro* sensitivity tests

D for pyogenic infections should only be altered after a trial of at least one week

E may best be a single broad-spectrum drug when bacteriological services are not available

10.4 **The following organisms are usually sensitive to the drugs quoted:**

A Gram-negative bacilli to benzylpencillin

B Spirochaetes to benzylpenicillin

C Staphylococci to gentamicin

D Chlamydia to tetracylines

E Strict anaerobes to metronidazole

+ve } cocci
-ve }
g+ve bacilli

10.5 **Bacterial resistance to antibiotics can arise**

A when naturally sensitive strains are eliminated, allowing naturally resistant organisms to proliferate

B from spontaneous mutation

C when sexual intercourse between cells allows the passage of plasmids

D by passage of bacteriophage from one cell to another

E by incorporation of DNA from lysed cells directly into bacteria

10.6 **Consequences of antibiotic use include**

A masking of infection

B arrest of synthesis of vitamin K by intestinal bacteria

C an intestinal malabsorption syndrome

D promotion of opportunistic infection

E candidiasis which is preventable by routine incorporation of nystatin in oral formulations

10.7 Combination of antibiotics should be used

A to delay development of drug resistance e.g. in tuberculosis

B to obtain synergism as in the case of penicillin and gentamicin in enterococcal endocarditis

C because if one drug is good, two can be counted on to be better

D to broaden the spectrum of antibacterial activity when infection is known to be mixed

E if a bacteristatic drug alone is thought to be insufficient, in which case a bactericidal drug should be added

10.8 Chemoprophylaxis is justified

A to prevent recurrent attacks of rheumatic fever

B to prevent recurrence of acute glomerulonephritis

C in epidemics of meningococcal meningitis

D to prevent bacterial endocarditis after dental procedures

E to prevent gas gangrene after mid-thigh amputation

10.9 The following statements about folic acid metabolism are correct:

A Folic acid is necessary for the formation of DNA and RNA

B Streptococci utilise preformed folate to form nucleic proteins

C Man is obliged to synthesise folate from para-aminobenzoic acid

D Organisms that are insensitive to sulphonamides are those that need to synthesise their own folic acid.

E Sulphonamides compete with para-aminobenzoic acid in the metabolic process with leads to folate

10.10 The combination of sulphonamide with trimethoprim

A is effective because successive enzymic reactions in the formation of folic acid are inhibited

B is safe because neither reaction which is inhibited occurs in man

C can cause macrocytic anaemia which may be successfully treated with folinic acid without inhibiting the therapeutic antibacterial effect

D is bactericidal although the individual drugs are bacteristatic

E commonly leads to drug resistance

10.11 Sulphonamides

A are generally more soluble in an alkaline urine

B achieve higher concentration in the blood than in the urine

C are more active after metabolism to the acetylated form

D are generally more active in an alkaline urine

E may precipitate in the urine to cause crystalluria

10.12 The following statements about sulphonamides are correct:

A Sulphadoxine has a long t½

B Salicylazosulphapyridine is principally used for urinary tract infections

C Phthalylsulphathiazole is poorly absorbed from the gut

D Sulphacetamide is suitable for topical use on the eye

E If allergic purpura occurs during treatment, the dose should be reduced for two or three days

10.13 Penicillins

A as a group have an identical range of antibacterial activity

B are only active against multiplying organisms

C may be less effective in the presence of tetracycline

D in all forms are resistant to degradation by gastric acid

E of the broad spectrum type (e.g. ampicillin) are adequate substitutes for benzylpenicillin

10.14 Among the principal organisms against which benzylpenicillin is used are

A pneumococci

B gonococci

C streptococci

D coliforms

E clostridia

10.15 Benzylpenicillin

A has a plasma t½ of about 3 hours
B is eliminated both by renal tubular secretion and by glomerular filtration
C competes with probenecid for elimination by the kidney
D should be given in frequent small doses to avoid excessive fluctuation in plasma concentration
E passes well through inflamed membranes

10.16 Allergies to penicillin

A may take the form of anaphylactic shock which can be fatal
B may be caused by degradation products as well as by penicillin itself
C can be relied on to disappear spontaneously with passage of time
D in healthy people should always be managed by an attempt at hyposensitisation
E can be predicted reliably and safely by skin testing

10.17 The following statements about penicillins are correct:

A Flucloxacillin taken orally is more fully absorbed and achieves higher blood concentration than is the case with oral cloxacillin
B Both flucloxacillin and cloxacillin are resistant to penicillinase
C Ampicillin and amoxycillin are destroyed by penicillinase (β-lactamase)
D Ampicillin is especially likely to cause a rash in patients with infectious mononucleosis
E Talampicillin is a form of ampicillin which has antibacterial activity only in the gut lumen

10.18 Cephalosporins

A are structurally dissimilar from penicillins in that they do not possess the beta-lactam ring

B were first obtained from a mould cultured from the sea near a Sardinian sewage outfall

C as a rule are excreted unchanged by the kidney

D penetrate well into brain and cerebrospinal fluid

E such as cephalexin and cephazolin do not appear in the bile

10.19 Cephalosporins

A in general are active against Gram-positive cocci

B in general are active against E. coli, Klebsiella and Proteus mirabilis

C may be nephrotoxic in high dose when combined with aminoglycosides

D may safely be used when there is a history of anaphylaxis to penicillin

E are useful for soft tissue infections caused by staphylococci and streptococci

10.20 The following statements about aminoglycoside antibiotics are correct:

A Aminoglycosides are generally inactivated by metabolism in the liver

B Aminoglycosides are batericidal because they bind to ribosomes causing incorrect aminoacid sequences to be entered into peptide chains

C Streptomycin instilled into visceral cavities may cause neuromuscular block

D Gram-negative bacilli are generally insensitive to aminoglycosides

E Plasmid-mediated transfer of genetic information may lead to the appearance of organisms resistant to several aminoglycosides

10.21 **The following statements about aminoglycoside antibiotics are correct:**

A In patients with renal failure blood concentration measurements and nomograms should be used as a guide to dosing

B Gentamicin should never be used in combination with benzylpenicillin

C Aminoglycosides transfer readily from blood to cerebrospinal fluid

D Ototoxicity with gentamicin affects the auditory rather than the vestibular portion of the eighth cranial nerve

E Neomycin is best reserved for systemic use

10.22 **Streptomycin**

A should be used alone in treating tuberculosis

B is more likely to be ototoxic in patients over the age of 40 years

C crosses the placenta and is potentially ototoxic to the fetus

D induced ototoxicity may be detected by caloric tests before serious symptoms occur

E treatment is free from allergic reactions

10.23 **Chloramphenicol**

A may be useful in severe H. influenzae meningitis

B is a drug of choice for bronchitis because of its effectiveness against H. influenzae

C causes aplastic anaemic in about one in 50 000 courses

D causes marrow depression which may be dose-related

E causes 'grey syndrome' in infants due to failure of the immature liver to conjugate the drug

10.24 **Tetracyclines**

A may damage the teeth of the fetus if given to a mother who is more than 14 weeks pregnant

B are actively transported into bacterial but not into human cells, which property confers selectivity of action.

C are active against Mycoplasma pneumoniae

D other than minocycline and doxycycline are eliminated by the kidney

E should be administered with milk to ensure optimal absorption

10.25 Tetracyclines can cause

A acute fatty liver of pregnancy

B decreased susceptibility to dental caries

C photosensitization

D suprainfection with yeasts or moulds

E serious growth disorder in children with chronic respiratory disease

10.26 The following statements about antibiotics are correct:

A Erythromycin is probably the most effective agent against the organism of Legionnaires' disease

B Erythromycin is useful to treat infection with Mycoplasma pneumoniae

C Vancomycin is the agent of choice for staphylococcal ileocolitis

D Clindamycin is the drug of choice for pseudomembranous enterocolitis

E Bacitracin should only be used parenterally

10.27 The following statements about antifungal drugs are correct:

A Nystatin is preferable to amphotericin B for systemic use

B Amphotericin B has a long plasma t½ and excretion of the drug continues for several weeks after administration has ceased

C Amphotericin may impair renal function

D Griseofulvin is a second-line drug for the treatment of candidiasis

E Griseofulvin prevents infection of new keratin but does not affect fungus already established

10.28 The following statements about antiviral drugs are correct:

A Idoxuridine should be applied in the early stage of herpes simplex ocular keratitis if it is to be effective

B Idoxuridine topically is valueless for cutaneous herpes zoster

C To prevent influenza A_2 infection amantadine should be taken continuously throughout the period of risk

D Patients who have received amantadine prophylactically develop antibodies to influenza A_2 and do not require subsequent immunisation

E Interferon is a natural host-defence substance

act- against penicillinase prod org

Methicillin
cloxicillin
cephalosporin
carbecillin
fusidic acid

11 Chemotherapy of Individual Diseases

11.1 The following statements about orally taken antimicrobials are correct:

A Erythromycin does not cause vomiting

B A high peak plasma concentration is more likely to be achieved if the drug is given before meals

C Relationship of dosing to meals is of little importance with cloxacillin

D PAS (sodium aminosalicylate) is ineffective if given on an empty stomach

E Potency is lost quicker in tropical than in temperate climates

11.2 Staphylococcal

A infections should be treated by a β-lactamase resistant penicillin if bacterial sensitivity tests are not available

B nasal carriers do not develop resistance to gentamicin in nasal cream

C skin carriers treated by concentrated hexachlorophane are at risk of central nervous system damage if they are infants

D pneumonia requires antimicrobial treatment for three weeks after the temperature has subsided

E enteritis is unresponsive to cloxacillin

11.3   In a case of streptococcal sore throat

A   local symptoms are well controlled by antimicrobial lozenges

B   sulphonamides are nearly as effective as penicillin in preventing late complications

C   immediate penicillin therapy should be given if there is a previous history of nephritis

D   if treatment with benzylpenillin is given it should ideally be continued for 10 days

E   local anaesthetic lozenges should be used to relieve discomfort in mild infections

11.4   Chemoprophylaxis of streptococcal infection

A   should be undertaken in all patients who have had an attack of nephritis

B   should be continued for life after a second attack of rheumatic fever

C   is especially important in the winter months

D   can be achieved by monthly penicillin injections as an alternative to oral treatment

E   entails some risk of endocarditis from penicillin-resistant Strept. viridans

11.5   Benzylpenicillin

A   readily controls Vincent's infection

B   has no part to play in the treatment of diphtheria

C   is dramatically effective in children under the age of 3 years suffering from whooping cough

D   is the drug of choice for Legionnaires' disease

E   is useful when given intrapleurally to a patient with empyema

11.6   In chronic bronchitis

A   it is essential to continue suppressive treatment throughout the year

B therapeutic trials have shown convincingly that ampicillin is superior to tetracycline as a suppressive drug

C expectorants are of little use

D an adrenal steroid can improve ventilation in some subjects

E if, in a patient on suppressive treatment, the sputum remains purulent, laboratory investigation is essential

11.7 In the therapy of infective endocarditis

A treatment should not be delayed once blood has been taken for culture, even if the organism has not been identified

B probenecid is especially useful in children

C Coxiella infections respond to vancomycin

D amphotericin B can be used with less risk of renal toxicity if combined with clotrimazole

E antimicrobial treatment should be continued as long as there is any clinical evidence of new emboli

11.8 An aminoglycoside

A is useful for providing antibiotic cover for dental extraction in patients with infective endocarditis already on therapeutic penicillin

B should be used together with penicillin in patients with infective endocarditis due to an unidentified organism

C is more likely to prove toxic in patients who are also taking probenecid

D is of little value in the treatment of septicaemic shock

E is bactericidal because it produces incorrect aminoacid sequences in intracellular peptide chains

11.9 In bacterial meningitis

A treatment should not be started before organisms have been recovered from the cerebrospinal fluid

B children with haemophilus infection should not be treated with both ampicillin and chloramphenicol because antagonism is likely

C due to steptococcus pneumoniae intrathecal treatment is essential for the first few days if ampicillin is used

D adrenal steroids should be used routinely to reduce inflammatory blocks in the subarachnoid space

E patients over 60 years of age are likely to be infected with Gram-negative gut bacteria

11.10 In the treatment of intestinal infections, the following statements are correct:

A Shigellosis, even if quite mild, demands urgent treatment with tetracycline

B Treatment of mild Salmonella infections with an antimicrobial drug is best avoided

C Campylobacter infections are often acquired from eating undercooked frozen chicken

D Metronidazole is the drug of choice for the treatment of post-operative anaerobic sepsis

E Both tetracycline and ampicillin are concentrated in bile

11.11 Suppression of bowel flora

A by oral antimicrobial drugs for two to three days before colonic surgery is mandatory

B in patients with a combination of hepatic and renal failure is best achieved by giving kanamycin

C is undesirable in the blind-loop syndrome

D may result in fatal pseudomembranous colitis

E by neomycin causes diarrhoea which is partly due to impairment of intestinal lactase activity

11.12 In the tratment of urinary tract infections

A an acid pH enhances the effect of chloramphenicol

B aminoglycosides can be used freely in the presence of renal failure

C   nitrofurantoin is as effective in pyelonephritis as in lower tract infection

D   nalidixic acid is active against proteus

E   methenamine is only used in chronic or recurrent infections when other drugs have failed

11.13 Isoniazid

A   is more effective against Myco. tuberculosis than is streptomycin

B   acts as efficiently in fast acetylators as in slow acetylators if given daily

C   is more likely to cause peripheral neuropathy in slow acetylators

D   is less likely to cause peripheral neuropathy if pyridoxine is also given

E   cannot be given intrathecally

11.14 Rifampicin

A   can attack intracellular bacilli because it is lipid soluble

B   loses its antibacterial activity after deacetylation in the liver

C   should be stopped at once if raised liver enzyme levels in the plasma are detected

D   causes harmless red discolouration of the urine

E   is more likely to cause immunologically mediated adverse reactions if the patient omits to take the drug on occasions

11.15 Ethambutol

A   is active against a wide range of bacterial species

B   does not need to be used in combination with other drugs

C   is more hepatotoxic than pyrazinamide

D   may cause monocular loss of visual acuity, so eyes should be tested separately

E   only passes into the cerebrospinal fluid in significant amounts if the meninges are inflamed

11.16 The following statements about antituberculosis treatment are correct:

A Triple drug therapy should be given until the results of sensitivity tests are known

B 'Short-course' chemotherapy (less than 18 months) has proved uniformly ineffectual

C The chances of success of once weekly regimes incorporating isoniazid are greater with slow acetylators

D Tuberculosis of the skin usually resists chemotherapy

E Adrenal steroids have a useful role in the treatment of severely ill patients

11.17 In eye infections

A superficial infections are best treated with sulphacetamide drops

B hydrocortisone can delay healing of corneal ulcers

C trachoma only responds to systemic treatment

D idoxuridine is sometimes of value in herpes simplex infections

E due to a virus hydrocortisone may make the condition worse

11.18 Tetracycline is the drug of choice for the treatment of

A pharyngeal gonorrhoea

B secondary syphilis

C non-gonococcal urethritis due to Chlamydia

D lymphogranuloma venereum

E granuloma inguinale

11.19 The following statements are correct:

A Treponema pallidum never becomes resistant to penicillin

B Trichomonas vaginitis responds less well to metronidazole if gonorrhoea is also present

C Vaginal candidiasis always responds satisfactorily to nystatin pessaries

D There is no effective treatment for non-specific vaginitis

E Podophyllin, though useful for plantar warts, is of no value in the treatment of genital warts

11.20 Benzylpenicillin is the best antimicrobial drug for

A skin sepsis in smallpox

B brucellosis

C gas gangere

D actinomycosis

E penetrating wounds of the chest

11.21 In acute amoebic dysentery

A metronidazole is the drug of choice

B the use of emetine is no longer thought to damage the myocardium

C there is no purpose in giving diloxanide at any stage of treatment

D tetracycline is beneficial in severe cases

E death is usually due to fluid and electrolyte loss

11.22 In the treatment of malaria

A primaquine acts on the hepatic cycle of the plasmodia

B suppressive treatment is designed to destroy the sporozoites injected by the mosquito

C chloroquine is of little use in treating a clinical attack

D prophylaxis against resistant strains in South East Asia is best undertaken with a combination of pyrimethamine and sulphadoxine

E quinine no longer has a significant part to play

11.23 The following statements are correct:

A Chloroquine is of some value in rheumatoid arthritis
B Prolonged administration of chloroquine can result in serious retinal toxicity
C Quinine may be useful in the treatment of nocturnal muscle cramps
D Quinine has no deleterious effect on visual acuity
E Proguanil, being loosely bound to plasma protein, only needs to be given once a week as a prophylactic against malaria

11.24 Metronidazole

A is superior to suramin in the treatment of African trypanosomiasis
B has no part to play in the control of leprosy
C has displaced pentamidine in the treatment of kala-azar
D is preferred to mepacrine in cases of giardiasis
E can produce a disulfiram-like effect with alcohol

11.25 The following statements about anthelmintics are correct:

A Piperazine causes neuromuscular block in the worm so that it is removed by normal peristaltic activity of the host
B Mebendazole is less toxic than tetrachloroethylene in ankylostomiasis
C Diethylcarbamazine is more effective against Onchocerca volvulus than against other filariae
D Thiabendazole controls muscular symptoms in trichiniasis
E If pyrantel is used in the treatment of a patient with enterobiasis, it is not necessary to treat the rest of the family in order to prevent reinfection

12 Corticotrophin, Adrenal Steroids and Antagonists

12.1 **The naturally occurring physiologically important secretions of the adrenal cortex include**

A cortisone
B hydrocortisone *(cortisol)*
C prednisolone
D aldosterone
E androgens

cortisol
Hydrocort
corticosterone

c̄ ACTH
↓ osteoporosis
↓ ms wasting
↓ Bruising
↓ Gastric upset
↓ Peptic ulcer
↓ gr wt, arrest
↑ Acne
↑ Hypertn

12.2 **The following statements about natural corticotrophin are correct:**

A It is a polypeptide consisting of 39 aminoacids
B Its biological activity resides in the first 24 aminoacids
C Its immunological antigenic activity resides in the final 15 aminoacids
D It has a plasma t½ of 3 hours *15*
E The response of the adrenal cortex to a rise in plasma corticotrophin begins after 30 minutes

12.3 **Natural corticotrophin**

A is active when taken by mouth
B is the major controlling factor in hydrocortisone production by the adrenal cortex
C is the major controlling factor in aldosterone production by the adrenal cortex
D is a preferred treatment for Addison's disease (primary adrenocortical insufficiency)
E is a preferred treatment for secondary adrenocortical insufficiency (hypopituitarism)

12.4 Tetracosactrin

A   is a synthetic polypeptide
B   has an aminoacid structure identical with natural corticotrophin
C   is more liable to induce immunological adverse reactions (allergy) than is corticotrophin obtained from animals
D   has a plasma t½ much longer than natural corticotrophin
E   is active when taken by mouth

12.5 Corticoliberin (corticotrophin releasing hormone, CRH)

A   is secreted by the hypothalamus in response to changing plasma concentrations of hydrocortisone
B   secretion is unaffected by environmental stress
C   secretion is unaffected by prednisolone administered for anti-inflammatory or immunosuppressive purposes
D   production is suppressed less during therapy with corticotrophin than with synthetic corticosteroids
E   is released in response to insulin hypoglycaemia and thus can be used in the diagnosis of Cushing's syndrome

12.6 In choosing between corticotrophin and a synthetic corticosteroid for therapy of asthma, account should be taken of the following:

A   Muscle wasting and osteoporosis are more likely with corticotrophin
B   Acne and hypertension are more likely with corticotrophin
C   Sudden withdrawal of therapy and intercurrent illness are less hazardous with corticotrophin
D   Adrenocortical atrophy is more prominent with synthetic corticosteroids
E   Growth suppression in children is a serious problem with corticotrophin

Biological ment

12.7 The following corticosteroids are pro-drugs:

A   Hydrocortisone
B   Cortisone — _is Prodrug & is conv. in vivo to Hydro cort_

C Prednisone
D Prednisolone
E Methylprednisolone

12.8 **The following statements about adrenocortical steroids are correct:**

A The actions of adrenocortical steroids are classified as mineralocorticoid and glucocorticoid
B Mineralocorticoid actions principally enhance sodium excretion and potassium retention
C Glucocorticoid actions principally affect metabolism of carbohydrate, protein and fat
D Glucocorticoid actions include suppression of inflammation and of immune responses
E Systemic administration of substantial doses induces suppression of the hypothalamic-pituitary-adrenocortical system via a feedback mechanism

12.9 **The following corticosteroids have largely or exclusively glucocorticoid actions:**

A Dexamethasone
B Hydrocortisone
C Fludrocortisone
D Prednisolone
E Cortisone

12.10 **An adrenal cortex suppressed by administration of a high therapeutic dose of adrenocortical steroid**

A continues to secrete androgen
B continues to secrete aldosterone
C will recover independently of hypothalamic-pituitary function
D puts the patient at hazard due to intercurrent disease
E puts the patient at hazard from forgetfulness

12.11 The following statements about the quantitative aspects of adrenocortical steroid function and therapy are correct:

A The normal daily secretion of hydrocortisone is 15 to 25 mg which is equivalent to 4 to 6 mg prednisolone for glucocorticoid effect

B Fifteen mg prednisolone administered daily will induce substantial suppression of the adrenal cortex

C High doses of corticosteroid induce clinically important suppression of the hypothalamic-pituitary-adrenocortical axis in less than one week

D Recovery of hypothalamic-pituitary-adrenocortical function is complete one week after withdrawal of a suppressive dose of corticosteroid

E Serious adverse effects are in general unlikely if the daily dose of corticosteroid is less than 15 mg prednisolone

12.12 Adrenocortical steroids are used

A as replacement therapy in adrenocortical insufficiency

B to suppress bacterial inflammation and antibody formation in shock

C in acute polyneuritis

D to suppress immunological inflammation

E to suppress the rejection of transplanted organs

12.13 The following statements about adrenocortical steroid therapy are correct:

A Atrophy of the adrenal cortex in long-term treatment is due to a direct effect on the hypothalamus

B There are no differences in the incidence of adverse effects with the principal corticosteroids

C Therapy should be stopped immediately an adverse effect appears

D Serious systemic adverse effects of topical (e.g. to skin) therapy are less likely with fluorinated than with non-fluorinated corticosteroids

E Sometimes a corticosteroid is given with the intention of suppressing (inhibiting) the hypothalamic-pituitary-adrenal axis

12.14 **Replacement therapy with corticosteroid**

A is best conducted with hydrocortisone because it has both mineralocorticoid and glucocorticoid effects

B is devised to mimic the pattern of natural hormone secretion during day and night

C is conducted at higher doses than pharmacotherapy

D may require added salt for optimal effect

E usually includes a small dose of fludrocortisone

12.15 **In long-term corticosteroid therapy for anti-inflammatory effect (pharmacotherapy)**

A prednisone is especially useful as it is not a pro-drug

B triamcinolone is liable to cause muscle wasting

C prednisolone is preferable to hydrocortisone because prednisolone has selective glucocorticoid actions

D cortisone is the drug of choice in patients with liver damage

E a weekly injection of corticotrophin should be given to prevent cortical atrophy

12.16 **The following statements about synthetic corticosteroids are correct:**

A They have a plasma t½ of 1-3 hours

B Their t½ is unaffected by liver disease or hepatic enzyme induction

C Alterations to plasma protein binding due to disease or other drugs may cause misleading results in laboratory tests eg for Cushing's syndrome

D Serious adverse effects such as osteoporosis may occur with as few as two doses

E In long term therapy the minimum effective dose should be used

12.17 Intermittent or alternate-day dosage with adrenocortical steroids

A minimizes hypothalamic-pituitary-adrenocortical suppression

B may be useful in replacement therapy for adrenocortical insufficiency

C is worth trying when immunosuppression is the objective

D is of particular value in rheumatoid arthritis

E reduces the risk of growth suppression in children

12.18 Long term adrenocortical steroid therapy carries an extra risk of adverse effects in patients giving a history of

A mental disorder

B peptic ulcer

C hypertension

D tuberculosis

E diabetes

12.19 Active immunization of patients taking long term corticosteroid therapy (for suppression of inflammation or immune responses)

A should never be attempted in children

B is hazardous with a killed vaccine

C is hazardous with a live vaccine

D is hazardous with a toxoid vaccine

E may be ineffective if the dose of corticosteroid is high

12.20 If a patient on long term corticosteroid therapy (whether for replacement or pharmacotherapy) develops an intercurrent illness, he should

A omit the next dose

B inform his doctor

C take large doses of oral potassium

D save a specimen of urine for the doctor to test

E post his 'steroid card' to the Department of Health and Social Security

12.21 Precautions to be taken during high dose long term corticosteroid therapy include

A regular weighing

B regular blood pressure measurement

C a regular urine test for sugar

D carrying a special card recording the details of treatment

E paying serious attention to any illness, however slight

12.22 Adverse effects of long-term corticosteroid therapy include

A osteoporosis

B hypertension

C muscle wasting

D deficient blood coagulation

E easy bruising

12.23 A patient who has taken corticosteroids for a long time may develop

A psychotic reactions

B pathological sleepiness

C menstrual disorders

D major skin damage after quite minor injury

E raised intracranial pressure

12.24 Long-term corticosteroid treatment may lead to

A hypothyroidism

B serious delayed tissue healing after surgery

C increased severity of infections

D masking of infections, which may produce atypical clinical features

E activation of dormant infections

12.25 Prolonged administration of corticosteroids causes

A oedema
B peptic ulcer
C glaucoma
D diabetes mellitus
E acne

12.26 The following statements about withdrawing adrenocorticosteroid pharmacotherapy that has lasted for many weeks are correct:

A The patient is at risk of acute adrenal insufficiency because the adrenal cortex has atrophied
B The longer the duration of therapy, the slower must be the withdrawal
C Corticotrophin should always be given to hasten recovery of the adrenal cortex
D If a patient cannot take the dose orally there should be no hesitation in using an injectable (i.m.) preparation
E If a patient requires surgery, even one year after withdrawal, a careful scheme of corticosteroid administration is required

12.27 The following statements about adrenocortical hormone synthesis and function are correct:

A Spironolactone is a competitive antagonist of aldosterone
B Metyrapone blocks corticosteroid receptors
C Metyrapone interferes with the enzymic synthesis of hydrocortisone
D Metyrapone can be used as a test for the capacity of the hypothalamic-pituitary axis to produce corticotrophin
E Spironolactone antagonises the therapeutic effect of carbenoxolone

13 Sleep, Hypnotics, Sedatives, Antiepileptics

13.1 A substance which

A induces drowsiness, sleep or stupor especially with analgesia is called a *narcotic*

B induces sleep is called a *hypnotic*

C calms and soothes without inducing sleep is called a *sedative*

D allays anxiety without materially impairing consciousness is called a *tranquillizer*

E has antipsychotic effect may be called a *neuroleptic*

13.2 The following statements about sleep are correct:

A Normal sleep is of two kinds

B The kinds of sleep may be characterised by eye movement patterns or electroencephalographic patterns

C Hypnotic-induced sleep is indistinguishable from normal sleep

D Normal sleep patterns are resumed immediately on withdrawal of a hypnotic after a period of continuous use

E All hypnotics can induce dependence

13.3 The following statements about hypnotics are correct:

A If a patient does not feel a hangover after a hypnotic he can count on his psychomotor performance being normal

B Hypnotics are best taken one hour before going to bed

C After a long period of continuous use a hypnotic should be withdrawn slowly over weeks.

D Where a patient objects to withdrawal so strongly that it is impracticable a benzodiazepine is the hypnotic of choice

E Barbiturates are never a first choice as a hypnotic

13.4 In treating insomnia

A Prescription of a hypnotic is not justified to help a patient through a sudden distressing situation, e.g. bereavement, as it is just this sort of use that carries risk of dependence

B prescription of a hypnotic is the first choice if the insomnia is chronic

C it is important to make a detailed enquiry into its cause and pattern

D it should be remembered that sleep requirement becomes less with increasing age

E benzodiazepines are the first choice as hypnotics

13.5 Benzodiazepines

A alter sleep pattern more than do other hypnotics

B are potent inducers of hepatic drug metabolizing enzymes

C are safer if taken in overdose than are other hypnotics

D do not have pharmacologically active metabolites

E should never be given to children

13.6 Barbiturates

A have a low therapeutic index

B are all more easily eliminated with the aid of alkaline diuresis

C are potent inducers of hepatic drug metabolizing enzymes

D cause only mild physical dependence

E which appear in glomerular filtrate are not reabsorbed in the renal tubule

13.7 The following statements about hypnotics and sedatives are correct:

A Paraldehyde, subjected to light and heat, decomposes to acetic acid

B Paraldehyde dissolves plastic syringes

C Chloral hydrate is a pro-drug

D Bromides still have a place in the treatment of nymphomania and spermatorrhoea

E Chlormethiazole is a hypnotic and sedative particularly advocated in alcoholism and the aged

13.8 In the management of overdose by hypnotics
A identification of the drug is not important
B active measures to eliminate the drug from the body are mandatory
C analeptics play a major role
D the objective is to restore the patient to full consciousness as quickly as possible
E mechanically assisted respiration plays a major role in severe cases

13.9 The life-endangering complications of hypnotic poisoning include
A fluid and electrolyte upset
B respiratory failure
C circulatory failure
D renal failure
E pneumonia

13.10 In the management of epilepsy
A all hypnotics and sedatives are useful
B patients must be persuaded of the importance of continuous medication
C treatment must be life long
D it may be possible to discover and eliminate precipitating factors
E the timing of medication should be adjusted if fits occur only at a particular time of day or night

13.11 In the management of epilepsy

A sudden cessation of treatment may result in status epilepticus

B monitoring plasma concentration of drugs is solely a research tool

C the majority of patients can be controlled on a single drug

D the physician needs to know and use the pharmacokinetic properties of each drug he prescribes

E long term drug therapy should be instituted after the first fit

13.12 In epileptic women under treatment

A there is a threefold increase in the rate of malformations in their children

B drug therapy should be stopped while they seek to become pregnant

C drug therapy should be stopped during pregnancy

D any malformation in their children is more likely to be due to the disease rather than the drugs

E the metabolism of oral contraceptives may be enhanced and a high dose oestrogen preparation should be used

13.13 In the treatment of epilepsy

A phenytoin is a first-choice drug for major seizures

B sodium valproate and ethosuximide are first-choice drugs for minor seizures

C paraldehyde is the first-choice drug for status epilepticus

D when the dose is changed some drugs may take a week or more to reach a steady concentration in the plasma

E adjustments of dosage can reliably be carried out by counting the frequency of fits

13.14 Phenytoin

A plasma $t\frac{1}{2}$ is the same at all plasma concentrations

B is subject only to first order kinetics

C enhances its own metabolism

D is unlikely to cause drug interactions in a patient taking other medication

E has a remarkably small range of adverse effects

13.15 The following statements about antiepileptic drugs are correct:

A   Sodium valproate is a potent hepatic enzyme inducer

B   In a patient taking sodium valproate blood coagulation should be examined before surgery is undertaken

C   Carbamazepine can be of value in epilepsy even if the patient does not suffer from trigeminal neuralgia as well

D   Clonazepam is of use in all principal forms of epilepsy

E   Troxidone, though safe, is obsolescent because of low efficacy

13.16 In tetanus prophylaxis

A   human tetanus immunoglobulin should be given to all patients with dirty wounds

B   a dose of human tetanus immunoglobulin gives reasonable protection for 4 weeks

C   injured subjects not known to be actively immune to tetanus should be given a dose of toxoid when seen, as the first dose of a course to be completed later

D   toxoid and immunoglobulin (antitoxin) may be mixed in the same syringe

E   a booster dose of toxoid is not necessary if the wounded subject has had a full course of toxoid (or a booster dose to a full course) within the past 10 years

13.17 In clinical tetanus

A   human immunoglobulin is of no value unless given intravenously

B   penicillin will not stop further production of toxin

C   tetanus spasms may be controlled by diazepam

D   chlorpromazine in large doses may make convulsions worse

E   treatment with tubocurarine and artificial respiration should be considered where spasms can otherwise only be controlled by making the patient unconscious

14 General Anaesthetics, Neuromuscular Blocking Agents, Local Anaesthetics

14.1   The following statements about stages of anaesthesia are correct:

A   In Stage I a sense of touch is retained and sense of hearing increased

B   In Stage 2 delirium precedes unconsciousness

C   In surgical anaesthesia (Stage 3) the corneal reflex does not disappear until plane IV

D   Some degree of medullary paralysis occurs at all planes of Stage 3

E   Stages 1 and 2 are hardly recognisable with modern techniques

14.2   The responsibility of the anaesthetist

A   begins immediately before surgery when the patient arrives at the operating theatre

B   is concerned with the patient's physical but not psychological condition

C   requires that he be informed of all drugs the patient may be receiving

D   involves providing unconsciousness, analgesia and muscular relaxation with a single drug whenever this is possible

E   ceases when patient leaves the operating theatre

14.3   Anaesthetic premedication involves considerations of providing

A   sedation

B   amnesia

C   analgesia

D   stimulation of the autonomic nervous system
E   quick recovery after surgery

14.4   A typical anaesthetic for abdominal surgery includes

A   gradual induction by an inhaled agent
B   maintenance by an agent given intravenously
C   analgesia by increasing the concentration of the inhaled agent
D   muscular relaxation with tubocurarine
E   the provision of apparatus for mechanically assisted respiration

14.5   After an abdominal operation the anaesthetist

A   may need to use antagonists to neuromuscular blocking agents
B   must not leave the patient until he is conscious
C   plays a role in the relief of postoperative pain
D   should ensure that the cough reflex is fully suppressed
E   cannot be expected to prevent postoperative vomiting

14.6   The single-handed operator/anaesthetist

A   should avoid making the patient unconscious if possible
B   may employ 'dissociative' anaesthesia
C   may employ 'neuroleptanalgesia'
D   may employ paraldehyde for procedures where there is no pain e.g. endoscopy
E   can safely use ether

14.7 **The following statements about the kinetics of inhalation anaesthetics are correct:**

A   An agent that is highly soluble in blood, given at constant rate, provides a slow induction

B   An agent that is relatively insoluble in blood, given at constant rate, provides a fast induction

C   Nitrous oxide provides slow induction

D   Diffusion anoxia occurs particularly with nitrous oxide when the agent is withdrawn

E   Recovery from anaesthesia is fast if the agent is relatively insoluble in blood

14.8 **Intravenous anaesthetics**

A   provide slow induction

B   provide particularly quick recovery even after prolonged use

C   depend for their duration of effect on redistribution of drug in the body

D   depending on metabolism for their elimination can be expected to have a short duration of action

E   can cause loss of the arm if injected by mistake into the brachial artery

14.9 **The following statements about ether and nitrous oxide are correct:**

A   In ether overdose cessation of respiration occurs before cardiac arrest

B   Ether is highly lipid soluble and given alone provides a slow and unpleasant induction

C   After even prolonged ether anaesthesia the postoperative recovery period is not unpleasant

D   Nitrous oxide cannot alone maintain surgical anaesthesia

E   In obstetrics a self-administered mixture of nitrous oxide 80%, oxygen 20% provides efficient and safe analgesia

14.10 **Halothane**

A   provides quick induction and recovery

B   causes hypotension and cardiac dysrhythmias

C   may cause jaundice if given repeatedly in the course of a few weeks

D should not be used if previous use has been followed by unexplained fever

E does not induce hepatic drug metabolizing enzymes

14.11 Thiopentone

A provides singularly pleasant induction

B causes sudden apnoea if injected rapidly

C does not often cause laryngospasm

D has a plasma t½ of 2.5 minutes in the early phase of an injection

E has a plasma t½ of 2 hours after equilibration

14.12 Neuromuscular blocking drug action is

A by competition

B by depolarisation

C by blocking autonomic ganglia

D reversible by an anticholinesterase in the case of suxamethonium

E reversible by chlorpromazine in the case of tubocurarine

14.13 Neuromuscular blocking drugs

A are used to provide muscular relaxation with only light anaesthesia by central nervous system depressants

B carry no risk of awareness during surgery

C are sufficiently selective to allow spontaneous respiration to be maintained in many cases

D acting by competition are preferred for long procedures

E acting by depolarisation do not cause postoperative muscle pain

14.14 Neuromuscular blocking agents are useful in therapy of

A myasthenia gravis

B status epilepticus

C spastic paraplegia

D tetanus

E electroconvulsive therapy (ECT)

14.15 Centrally-acting muscle relaxants, e.g. baclofen

A are prone to cause objectionable sedation
B improve voluntary motor power
C may make the patient worse even if spasticity in the legs is reduced
D control flexor spasms
E require provision of artificial respiration

14.16 A desirable local anaesthetic should

A be non-irritant to tissues
B have a slow onset of action
C be soluble in water
D be sterilisable by heat
E have a built-in vasodilator action

14.17 Local anaesthetics

A act by altering ionic permeability of nerve cell membranes
B prevent initiation and propagation of the nerve impulse
C may be absorbed sufficiently to cause systemic toxicity
D affect first the larger (motor) nerve fibres and last the small (sensory) fibres
E are all absorbed across mucous membranes

14.18 Local anaesthetic

A action may be prolonged by addition of a vasodilator
B application to extremities (e.g. toe) should always be conducted with added adrenaline
C mixed with adrenaline may cause severe hypertension in a patient taking a monoamine oxidase inhibitor
D mixed with adrenaline may cause severe hypertension in a patient taking a tricyclic antidepressant
E mixed with felypressin is preferable in patients with cardiovascular disease

14.19   Local anaesthetics

A   are usually effective within 5 minutes of application
B   have a useful duration of action of 1-2 hours
C   are most stable in the form of acid salts
D   have an enhanced action in inflamed tissues
E   are absorbed and metabolized in the liver

14.20   Local anaesthetic

A   overdose can cause convulsions
B   overdose can cause cardiovascular collapse
C   may be applied to a surface
D   may be infiltrated around the lesion
E   must never be infiltrated around major peripheral nerves
     or near the spinal cord

14.21   Lignocaine

A   is useful in cardiac arrhythmias
B   is less toxic than prilocaine in overdose
C   unlike prilocaine, is not effective when applied to
     mucous membranes
D   differs structurally from most other local anaesthetics
E   carries no risk of convulsions in overdose

14.22   Cocaine

A   is effective on mucous membranes
B   enhances natural catecholamine effects
C   is well absorbed from mucous membranes
D   is abused for its central nervous system stimulation
E   overdose should be treated by adrenoceptor blocking
     drugs

14.23 **The following statements about the use of drugs in childbirth are correct:**

A   Pethidine depresses fetal respiration more than morphine

B   Naloxone antagonizes morphine but not pethidine

C   Nitrous oxide is a potent fetal respiratory depressant despite its brief action

D   Diazepam dose must be carefully restricted as it is capable of depressing the newborn baby for several days

E   Vasoconstrictors can cause fetal distress by reducing placental blood flow

14.24 **When drugs are used in childbirth**

A   it is important to work out a schedule of drug dosage in advance and not to be diverted from it

B   opiates delay gastric emptying

C   a dose of metoclopramide will ensure an empty stomach in a patient who has received pethidine, if general anaesthesia is needed

D   neuromuscular blocking agents must be avoided in Caesarian section

E   halothane does not enter the fetus

14.25 **The following statements about the interaction of anaesthetics with other drugs are correct:**

A   A patient taking a monoamine oxidase inhibitor may be premedicated with morphine

B   A patient under treatment for hypertension is liable to hypotension during general anaesthesia

C   Oral contraceptives predispose to postoperative thrombo-embolism

D   Diuretic-induced hypokalaemia potentiates neuromuscular blocking drugs

E   Aminoglycoside antibiotics antagonize neuromuscular blocking drugs

14.26 **Special care before and during general anaesthesia is required in patients having**

A mitral stenosis
B renal failure
C myasthenia gravis
D porphyria
E diabetes mellitus

14.27 **Factors which may influence the normal response to anaesthesia include**

A hypothyroidism
B malignant hyperpyrexia
C sickle-cell trait
D the age of the patient
E atmospheric pollution of the operating theatre

14.28 **In premedication**

A morphine is particularly dangerous in cases of raised intracranial pressure
B benzodiazepines are best avoided in anxious patients
C hyoscine can cause confusion in the old
D pethidine is preferable to morphine in asthmatics
E atropine may precipitate glaucoma even in a single dose of less than 1 mg

15 Analgesics, Pain, Rheumatism

15.1 **The following statements about testing of analgesic drugs are correct:**

A Placebos give relief in about 35% of cases
B Emotional respose to pain can largely be ignored in volunteer experiments
C Double-blind technique is unnecessary
D Animal experiments are valueless
E The sex of the observer may affect the response of the patient to analgesics

15.2 **Pain**

A from visceral smooth muscle responds best to aspirin
B from spasm of striated muscle should first be treated with an opiate
C of thalamic origin may respond to chlorpromazine
D of trigeminal neuralgia should in the first instance be treated with pentazocine
E of inflammation responds to aspirin

15.3 **In migraine**

A vasoactive amines in the diet may play a part in causing an attack
B propranolol can be effective in prophylaxis
C an acute attack should be treated with clonidine
D methysergide is a drug of last resort because of the risk of retroperitoneal fibrosis
E clonidine may be of value for prophylaxis

15.4 Ergotamine

- **A** is valuable for preventing migraine
- **B** in overdose can cause gangrene of the extremities
- **C** is safe to use in pregnancy
- **D** is best avoided in obliterative vascular disease
- **E** is most effective if given early in an attack of migraine

15.5 Endorphins

- **A** are naturally-occurring peptides
- **B** counteract the analgesic activity of morphine
- **C** are endogenously regulated
- **D** are not neurotransmitters
- **E** probably play an important role in the phenomena of opiate dependence and withdrawal

15.6 Morphine can cause

- **A** miosis
- **B** convulsions in overdose
- **C** biliary tract spasm
- **D** antidiuresis
- **E** sleep

15.7 Morphine should if possible be avoided in patients with

- **A** pancreatitis
- **B** asthma
- **C** respiratory depression
- **D** paroxysmal nocturnal dyspnoea
- **E** ureteric colic

15.8   Morphine may safely be given

A   subcutaneously to shocked patients
B   in small doses to patients with hepatic failure
C   in small doses to control diarrhoea
D   together with a monoamine oxidase inhibitor
E   repeatedly to patients with trigeminal neuralgia

15.9   Morphine and heroin dependence

A   are more disabling socially and physically than is opium dependence
B   should be treated by abrupt withdrawal of the drug
C   are acceptable in the management of chronic pain in the terminally ill
D   can occur within 24 hours if the drug is given 4-hourly
E   can occur in infants born to addicted mothers

15.10   The following statements about opiates are correct:

A   Codeine is as effective an analgesic as is morphine
B   Codeine in large doses causes excitement
C   Codeine is partly converted to morphine in the body
D   Pethidine does not constrict the pupils
E   Pethidine does not suppress cough usefully

15.11   The following statements about opiates are correct:

A   Dependence induced by methadone is less severe than that induced by morphine
B   Heroin is useful for cough in the dying
C   Weight for weight heroin is a more effective inducer of dependence than is morphine
D   Pentazocine does not induce dependence
E   Naloxone does not antagonise the actions of pentazocine

15.12   The following statements are correct:

A   Dextropropoxyphene is safer than codeine in large doses

B Fentanyl has a longer duration of action than has morphine

C Naloxone can be used to reveal opiate dependence

D Naloxone antagonises the action of nefopam

E Fentanyl is used for neuroleptanalgesia

15.13 In the patient terminally ill with cancer

A local radiotherapy may relieve pain due to nerve entrapment

B headache due to raised intracranial pressure responds to dexamethasone

C anorexia may be helped by prednisolone

D prostaglandin synthetase inhibitors are effective for bone pain due to metastases

E and in continuous pain the interval between doses of analgesics should be short enough to prevent pain recurring

15.14 Non-steroidal anti-inflammatory drugs

A with least anti-inflammatory action are as a rule most toxic.

B may have negligible intrinsic analgesic activity

C stimulate prostaglandin degradation

D may be used to close patent ductus arteriosus in the newborn

E do not give rise to serious dependence

15.15 Paracetamol

A is about equivalent to indomethacin in anti-inflammatory activity

B has a t½ of approximately 20 hours

C is metabolized in part to a highly reactive metabolite

D overdose should be treated with N-acetyl cysteine provided 12 hours have elapsed since paracetamol was taken

E is about equivalent to aspirin in analgesic activity

15.16 Aspirin

A stimulates respiration
B in high doses causes metabolic acidosis in children
C in doses of less than 2 g per day causes urate retention
D inhibits sweating
E shortens prothrombin time

15.17 Aspirin

A when taken regularly causes loss of about 5 ml of blood per day from the gastrointestinal tract
B when taken with alcohol has a greater risk of gastrointestinal haemorrhage than has aspirin on its own
C is poorly absorbed through the gastric mucosa
D in a single oral dose is probably mainly absorbed from the small intestine
E is metabolized by processes which may saturate at high therapeutic doses

15.18 Overdose with aspirin

A causes deafness
B causes respiratory alkalosis in adults
C may appropriately be treated by forced acid diuresis
D clinically resembles diabetic ketoacidosis
E may require treatment by haemodialysis

15.19 Phenylbutazone

A should be given three times daily to maintain steady plasma concentrations
B is unlikely to be involved in drug interactions by competition for protein binding sites
C induces hepatic enzymes
D causes salt and water retention
E has more marked analgesic than anti-inflammatory action

15.20 The following statements are correct:

A Indomethacin causes dizziness and lightheadedness

B Sulindac is itself inactive but is converted by metabolism to an active form

C Salicylates prevent the late cardiac complications of rheumatic fever

D A corticosteroid should be used instead of a salicylate in rheumatic fever with cardiac enlargement

E Salicylates commonly take more than one week to relieve pain and inflammation in acute rheumatism

15.21 In the treatment of rheumatoid arthritis

A regular measurements of plasma salicylate concentration are mandatory

B penicillamine is reserved for patients with active progressive disease, in whom anti-inflammatory analgesics have failed

C with penicillamine, if renal damage occurs, it will be permanent

D response to sodium aurothiomalate usually occurs within the first two weeks of treatment

E adverse effects of gold may be treated with dimercaprol

15.22 In the treatment of rheumatoid arthritis

A azathioprine has a useful corticosteroid-sparing effect

B systemic corticosteroids are particularly useful in the elderly disabled subject

C hydrocortisone has no part to play unless one joint is more severely affected than others

D with chloroquine, retinal damage may occur

E with chloroquine, bleaching of the hair may occur

15.23 In the treatment of gout

A colchicine may relieve pain and inflammation in a few hours

B probenecid may provoke an acute attack

C allopurinol is valuable because of its uricosuric action

D sulphinpyrazone acts by blocking the production of uric acid

E colchicine is an effective suppressant prophylactic

15.24 In the treatment of gout

A response to colchicine may help to make the diagnosis

B corticosteroids are contra-indicated

C salicylates should not be given concurrently with other uricosurics

D drugs that lower plasma urate should be discontinued after six months

E amiloride should be avoided

15.25 Analgesic abuse

A is associated with an increased incidence of renal pelvic tumours

B characteristically causes interstitial nephritis with renal papillary necrosis

C carries a greater risk of renal damage in diabetics than in non-diabetics

D causing renal damage is exclusively due to phenacetin

E causing nephropathy is commonly manifested by nocturia and renal colic

16 Non-medical Use of Drugs, Drug Dependence, Tobacco, Alcohol, Cannabis, etc.

16.1 The following statements about non-medical drug use and drug abuse are correct:

A Abuse potential of a drug is related to its capacity to produce immediate satisfaction

B Abuse potential of a drug is uninfluenced by its route of administration

C Drugs that insulate the individual from environmental stress and anxiety are the most likely to be abused

D Drugs that can provide an intense pleasurable experience are particularly likely to be abused

E Multiple drug abuse is common

16.2 The following statements about non-medical drug use or abuse are correct:

A Criteria for what constitutes drug abuse are the same for all societies

B It is not the drug alone, but also the way it is used that provides the basis for the classification 'hard' and 'soft'

C Spiritual or religious experience can be regarded as a normal dose-related pharmacodynamic effect of some drugs

D The claim that drugs can provide a basis for a 'culture' may best be judged by results, ie by the contribution of its exponents to society in terms of practice and example

E Even 'soft' use of drugs such as alcohol and tobacco is so potentially hazardous that it should be countered by legislation

16.3 **The following statements about the use of drugs to gain advantage in sport are correct:**

A Anabolic steroids are used by athletes to improve performance in the 100 metre sprint

B Amphetamines are used to improve performance in weight-lifting

C Detection of drug use is specially difficult where drug or metabolites are closely related to physiological substances

D Caffeine may be taken as diet (coffee) or as medicine (tablets)

E Caffeine can improve physical performance

16.4 **Features of the drug dependent state include**

A emotional distress if the drug is withheld

B physical illness if the drug is withheld

C a need to increase the dose

D continuous use

E intermittent use

16.5 **The following statements about drug dependence and tolerance are correct:**

A Physical dependence is a major factor with cocaine

B Physical dependence is a major factor with heroin

C Cross tolerance occurs between members of the same chemical class of drug

D Cross tolerance occurs between members of different chemical classes of drug

E Dependence is confined to drugs that alter consciousness

16.6 **The following statements about drug abuse are correct:**

A Young teenagers can purchase glues and aerosols without question from the vendor whereas the vendor of alcohol has a motive to refuse sale

B Heroin abuse occurs chiefly amongst teenagers

C Alcohol abuse occurs at all adult ages

D What a man may lawfully seek in wine surely he may lawfully find in opium

E Young users of drugs by the intravenous route have a mortality up to 40 × normal

16.7 Established opiate addicts

A of long standing take the drug *primarily* to avoid the unpleasantness of withdrawal

B who self-inject can easily be transferred to oral methadone since this preparation also provides the sought-after 'kick' or 'high'

C who are in pain from a physical injury can be treated satisfactorily by giving a different opiate in ordinary dose

D who self-inject are particularly liable to life-endangering infections and thromboembolism

E who have been subjected to complete drug withdrawal and have regained physical health are not specially prone to relapse

16.8 Morphine-type drug dependence is characterised by

A severe physical dependence

B slight emotional dependence

C marked tolerance

D cross-tolerance with other opiates

E resistance to naloxone

16.9 Barbiturate-type drug dependence is characterised by

A severe emotional dependence

B slight physical dependence

C tolerance

D cross-tolerance with alcohol

E cross-tolerance with benzodiazepines

16.10 **The following statements about drug abuse or dependence are correct:**

A   Cannabis induces marked physical dependence and tolerance
B   Tobacco induces severe emotional dependence
C   Amphetamine use, if prolonged, can cause a psychotic state
D   Cocaine induces marked tolerance
E   Drug mixtures, e.g. barbiturate-amphetamine, induce mood effects that do not occur with either drug alone

16.11 **The following statements about tobacco smoking are correct:**

A   Smoke of pipes and cigars is alkaline and therefore nicotine is readily absorbed via the buccal mucosa
B   Smoke of cigarettes is acidic and therefore nicotine is not readily absorbed via the buccal mucosa
C   Cigarette smokers tend to inhale
D   Cigar and pipe smokers tend not to inhale
E   Cigarette smokers who inhale may have as much as 15% of their haemoglobin converted to carboxyhaemoglobin

16.12 **The following statements about smoking are correct:**

A   Tobacco can be aptly described as 'a pharmacological aid in man's search for contentment'
B   Cigarette smokers tend to have introverted rigid personalities
C   Sigmund Freud suggested that a powerful motive for smoking might be persistence into adult life of a childhood 'constitutional intensification of the erotogenic significance of the labial region'
D   Sigmund Freud did not smoke
E   Starting to smoke may be linked with 'self-esteem and status needs'

16.13 Pharmacological factors involved in smoking include

A adjustment of plasma nicotine concentration by automatic changes in puffing rate and inhalation
B avoidance of nicotine withdrawal feelings
C a mix of sedative and stimulant action on the central nervous system depending on the psychological state at the time
D increased airways resistance
E no notable cardiovascular effects

16.14 The following statements about the risks of tobacco smoking are correct:

A 15% of male non-smokers aged 35 years are dead by age 65 years
B 40% of male smokers of 25 or more cigarettes are dead by age 65 years
C Cigarette smoking causes induction of hepatic metabolizing enzymes
D The extra death risk of smokers is not altered by stopping smoking
E The extra death rate of smokers is chiefly the result of cardiovascular and respiratory diseases

16.15 The risk of death from lung cancer is influenced by

A number of cigarettes smoked
B age of starting smoking
C use of filter-tipped cigarettes
D giving up smoking
E use of pipe or cigars

16.16 Smoking is a risk factor for

A coronary heart disease
B deep vein thrombosis
C bronchitis and emphysema
D peptic ulcer
E still-birth

16.17 The following statements about ethyl alcohol (ethanol) are correct:

A Absorption is almost confined to the stomach

B Food, especially milk, delays absorption

C Habitual drinkers metabolize alcohol more rapidly than non-habitual drinkers

D It is selectively stored in body fat

E It is subject to saturation or zero-order kinetics

16.18 Alcohol-dependence is characterised by

A slight emotional dependence

B trivial physical dependence

C inability to discuss the problem

D absence of tolerance

E surreptitious drinking

16.19 Alcohol characteristically causes

A loss of finer grades of judgement and attention even at low doses

B loss of power to control mood

C increase in physical efficiency

D peripheral vasoconstriction

E increased secretion of antidiuretic hormone

16.20 The following statements about alcohol are correct:

A Gastric acid secretion is first inhibited then increased

B After an initial increase in blood dextrose alcohol causes hypoglycaemia which can be severe

C Vomiting is primarily due to a direct gastric irritant action

D In acute overdose inhalation of vomit is the commonest cause of death

E Fetal damage occurs in pregnant alcoholics

16.21 Chronic alcohol dependence is characterised by

A psychotic states
B nutritional deficiences
C cholestatic hepatitis
D dementia
E recovery if the subject stops drinking, even at a late stage

16.22 Acute overdose of alcohol can cause

A excited and violent behaviour which is best controlled by a barbiturate given intramuscularly
B an episode of acute hepatitis in a chronic alcoholic who already has liver disease
C fall in serum transaminase
D hypolipidaemia
E hyperuricaemia and acute gout

16.23 Methyl alcohol (methanol)

A is sometimes drunk as a substitute for ethyl alcohol
B is metabolized to acetaldehyde
C causes intense acidosis
D overdose is treated by sodium bicarbonate and ethyl alcohol
E overdose may cause permanent blindness

16.24 The following statement about psychodysleptics and hallucinogens (lysergide or LSD, mescaline etc.) are correct:

A They have no proved therapeutic use
B Their actions cannot be described as precisely as is possible for most other drugs since their effects are highly conditioned by the subject's frame of mind, personality and environment
C They do not cause psychotic reactions
D Physical dependence occurs
E 'Bad trips' may be treated with diazepam

16.25   When cannabis is taken

A   tolerance does not occur
B   memory and attention are impaired and the subject becomes more suggestible
C   cannabinoids are taken up in body fat and slowly released
D   vasodilatation and tachycardia are usual
E   psychotic reactions do not occur

17 Drugs and Mental Disorder

17.1 Psychotropic drugs

- **A** act by modifying chemotransmitter systems in the nervous system
- **B** are more likely to be effective in neuroses than in psychoses
- **C** act in the reticular activating system which particularly influences arousal
- **D** act in the limbic system which particularly influences affect or emotion
- **E** act in the hypothalamus which particularly influences the autonomic system

17.2 Schizophrenic states

- **A** are particularly associated with dopaminergic activity in the brain
- **B** are benefited by drugs that block dopamine receptors
- **C** are benefited by the phenothiazine group of neuroleptics
- **D** manifesting themselves with negative symptoms, e.g. apathy, respond particularly well to drug therapy
- **E** manifesting themselves with positive symptoms, e.g. delusions, respond particularly poorly to drug therapy

17.3 Depressive states

A are particularly associated with cholinergic activity in the brain

B are benefited by drugs that block adrenoceptors in the brain

C respond to drugs after 7–14 days

D respond to electroshock treatment even more slowly than to drugs

E are currently best explained by changes in monoamine function in the brain

17.4 The following statements about mania are correct:

A Mania may be accompanied by overactivity of catecholamine transmission in the brain

B Lithium benefits mania by altering amine metabolism or receptor function

C Lithium should only be used in severe cases

D A phenothiazine neuroleptic is a drug of first choice for acute mania

E Phenothiazine neuroleptics block both dopamine and α-adrenoceptors

17.5 The following statements about anxiety are correct:

A Psychic anxiety responds particularly to β-adrenoceptor blocking drugs

B Somatic symptoms of anxiety respond particularly to an α-adrenoceptor blocking drug

C Anxiety manifested as either or both psychic or somatic manifestations responds to a benzodiazepine

D Benzodiazepines probably act by enhancing the effects of the natural inhibitor (in the nervous system) gamma-aminobutyric acid (GABA)

E Pre-examination panic in students cannot be benefited by drugs

17.6 The following statements about the management of depression are correct:

A For prevention of unipolar depression lithium is better than a tricyclic antidepressant

B For prevention of bipolar depression a tricyclic antidepressant is better than lithium
C If a drug fails then electroconvulsive therapy will also fail
D Most cases of depression recover spontaneously
E Amphetamine is useful in depression

17.7 Psychotropic drugs may be classified as

A neuroleptics
B anxiolytic sedatives
C antidepressants
D psychostimulants
E psychodysleptics

17.8 In psychiatry

A drug responses are easy to measure
B dosage of drug can be readily and precisely adjusted according to clinical response
C ideal therapeutic response may occur at intermediate plasma concentrations of some antidepressants
D where therapeutic response is difficult to measure it is particularly useful to know the plasma concentration of the drug
E dose increments should be added at intervals that take into account the half-life of the drug

17.9 Actions of neuroleptics include

A dopamine receptor block
B α-adrenoceptor block
C β-adrenoceptor block
D anticholinergic effects
E potentiation of other drugs

17.10 **Adverse reactions to phenothiazine neuroleptics include**

A cholestatic jaundice
B hypotension
C dry mouth
D parkinsonian syndrome
E tardive dyskinesia

17.11 **With injected (i.m.) long-acting depot neuroleptics**

A patient non-compliance is halved
B defaulters are identifiable
C hepatic first-pass metabolism is enhanced
D extrapyramidal syndromes are common and are treated by an anticholinergic drug
E severe depression can occur

17.12 **Benzodiazepines**

A are classified as anxiolytic sedatives
B only rarely induce dependence
C induce hepatic drug-metabolizing enzymes
D in overdose are particularly liable to cause respiratory depression
E can release suppressed aggression

17.13 **The following statements about tricyclic antidepressants are corrrect:**

A Cholinergic side-effects are common
B Interactions with sympathomimetics and antihypertensives are clinically important
C To reduce non-compliance it is particularly important to advise depressed patients of even relatively minor adverse effects
D Overdose carries serious cardiovascular hazard
E Overdose is readily treated by dialysis because they have a large apparent volume of distribution

17.14 Tricyclic antidepressants

A can be expected to relieve depression within 48 hours
B may be given in single evening dose
C have plasma t½s that may vary from 10–200 hours
D can be effective in nocturnal enuresis in children but are too dangerous to be used other than in exceptional circumstances
E are no use in chronic pain

17.15 When making a choice of antidepressant it is useful to take into account that

A amitriptyline has sedative effect
B imipramine has no sedative effect
C desipramine has stimulant effect
D mianserin is comparatively free from cardiotoxic effect
E mianserin does not antagonize antihypertensives

17.16 Monoamine oxidase inhibitors

A cause decrease in catecholamines and 5-hydroxytryptamine in the central nervous system
B allow increased absorption of monoamines from the gut
C allow reduced hepatic first-pass metabolism of monoamines absorbed from the gut
D potentiate injected sympathomimetics that act directly on adrenoceptors (e.g. adrenaline in local anaesthetic)
E potentiate injected sympathomimetics that act indirectly by causing release of noradrenaline stores

17.17 A patient on treatment with a monoamine oxidase inhibitor is at risk for a hypertensive reaction if he consumes

A milk
B yogurt
C butter
D cheese
E scrambled egg

17.18   From knowledge of the mechanism of hypertensive crisis in a patient taking a monoamine oxidase inhibitor it is evident that immediate control of the blood pressure will be achievable with

A   propranolol
B   methyldopa
C   captopril
D   clonidine
E   phentolamine

17.19   The following statements about lithium are correct:

A   Slow release formulation is useful
B   It is distributed throughout body water, ie its apparent volume of distribution is about 50 litres in a 70 kg person
C   Its use must be controlled by regular measurement of plasma concentration
D   In case of toxicity it is not readily dialysable
E   Its principal use is in prophylaxis of manic-depressive disorder

17.20   Amphetamine

A   acts by increasing the amount of noradrenaline stored in nerve endings throughout the nervous system
B   excites adults but sedates some hyperactive children
C   overdose can cause an acute psychotic state
D   overdose can cause hyperpyrexia
E   is useful in narcolepsy

17.21   The following statements about appetite suppressants are correct:

A   They are often sympathomimetics related to amphetamine
B   They are not subject to abuse and do not induce dependence
C   Fenfluramine (Ponderax) is related to amphetamine but acts via serotonin (5HT) rather than noradrenaline

D Fenfluramine antagonizes antihypertensive drugs

E They should be used only briefly as their effect is transient

17.22 The following statements about caffeine and caffeine-containing drinks are correct:

A Caffeine acts as a phosphodiesterase inhibitor, preventing destruction of cyclic AMP

B Caffeine has a t½ of 1 to 2 hours

C Clinically significant overdose of caffeine can occur with 12 cups of coffee or 5 cups of tea a day

D Caffeine overdose may mimic an anxiety state

E Theophylline has actions similar to caffeine

18 Cough, Respiratory Stimulants and Vomiting

18.1 Cough

A even if productive may require to be suppressed after eye surgery

B is reduced by a warm, moist atmosphere

C can be made less exhausting by mucolytics in some patients

D is reduced by opiates

E is little affected by psychogenic factors

18.2 Cough

A arising above the larynx may be benefited by water aerosol inhalation

B is relieved by antihistamines through block of histamine H_1-receptors

C arising below the larynx should be treated with syrups or lozenges that coat the mucosa

D may be improved by rehydrating a dehydrated patient

E is improved by atropine

18.3 The use of a respiratory stimulant

A is indicated in chronic ventilatory failure with hypercapnia

B is contraindicated as an emergency measure in respiratory depression due to drugs

C such as doxapram may reduce postoperative respiratory complications

D such as picrotoxin is dangerous because of the risk of convulsions

E such as aminophylline may be useful in apnoeic infants

18.4 Antiemetics

A that act on the emetic centre in the brain affect vomiting from any cause

B that act on the chemoreceptor trigger zone in the brain only affect vomiting mediated by chemoreceptor stimulation

C for motion sickness should only be given once nausea is experienced

D may intensify sedation due to alcohol

E such as hyoscine should be used for motion sickness on short journeys

18.5 Vomiting

A caused by morphine is due to stimulation of the gastrointestinal tract

B caused by digoxin is due to stimulation of the chemoreceptor trigger zone of the brain

C after anaesthesia can be reduced by chlorpromazine

D in pregnancy may be an indication for pyridoxine

E due to radiation responds to metoclopramide

18.6 Metoclopramide

A acts on the chemoreceptor trigger zone

B blocks dopaminergic receptors

C can be used to treat extrapyramidal dystonia

D is particularly useful for vomiting caused by cytotoxic drugs

E reduces gastric secretion

18.7   Therapeutic emesis

A   with ipecacuanha should cause vomiting within 20 minutes, lasting for less than 30 minutes

B   with ipecacuanha is due to both peripheral (stomach) and central (chemoreceptor trigger zone) actions

C   with ipecacuanha even in an emergency should only be undertaken by a doctor

D   with apomorphine is safe in the unconscious patient

E   is contraindicated when a corrosive substance has been swallowed

19 Cholinergic and Anticholinergic Drugs

19.1 **The following statements about cholinergic drugs are correct:**

A Atropine antagonises all the effects of cholinergic drugs except those at autonomic ganglia and the neuromuscular junction *[nicotinic]*

B Pilocarpine inhibits cholinesterase

C Physostigmine acts selectively on end-organs that respond to acetylcholine

D Carbachol has more prominent muscarinic than nicotinic effects

E Vasodilator effects of cholinergic drugs are mainly direct and are unrelated to cholinergic vasodilator nerves

[Blood vessels, Post ganglionic cholinergic → muscarinic Sweat gland]

19.2 **Cholinergic stimulation causes**

A intra-ocular pressure to rise

B lachrymation

C tachycardia

D bronchodilatation

E colicky abdominal pain

19.3 **The following statements are correct:**

A Carbachol is safe to give intravenously

B Bethanechol is an anticholinesterase

C Pilocarpine has a clinically useful miotic action

D Muscarinic effects are characteristic of poisoning with the fungus Amanita muscaria

E Severe hypoglycaemia may occur in poisoning with the fungus Amanita phalloides

19.4 The following statements are correct:

A Pseudocholinesterase enzymes are mainly present in nerve endings

B Organophosphorus anticholinesterases are usually competitive inhibitors of cholinesterase enzymes

C Pseudocholinesterases destroy esters other than acetylcholine e.g. procaine

D Atropine reverses all the adverse effects of anticholinesterase poisoning

E Pralidoxime functions by reactivating cholinesterase

19.5 In myasthenia gravis

A neostigmine given for diagnostic purposes should be accompanied by atropine to suppress unwanted visceral (muscarinic) effects

B if the daily dose of anticholinesterase is less than 15 tablets and the pupil diameter exceeds 3 mm, weakness is likely to be due to excess of cholinergic action

C weakness that increases more than two hours after a dose and is relieved by the next dose is probably myasthenic

D edrophonium exaggerates a myasthenic crisis and alleviates a cholinergic crisis

E habitual use of atropine may mask excessive therapy

19.6 In myasthenia gravis

A excessive parasympathetic activity indicates overdose of anticholinesterase

B overdose of drugs is probably one of the major causes of death

C a cholinergic crisis should be treated with parathion

D there is a reduced number of acetylcholine receptors at the neuromuscular junction

E thymectomy is usually advisable if a thymoma is present

19.7 Atropine

A inhibits milk production

B promotes sweating

C alters gastric pH

D relaxes smooth muscle
E lowers intra-ocular pressure in an eye predisposed to narrow-angle glaucoma

19.8 Atropine

A administration to the eye may interfere with normal pupillary reflexes for up to two weeks
B reduces the heart rate
C loosens sticky bronchial secretions
D opposes cholinergic activity at the neuromuscular junction
E prevents and suppresses motion sickness

19.9 In overdose atropine causes

A mydriasis
B hallucinations
C hypothermia
D coma
E dry mouth

19.10 Anticholinergic drugs may be used in the treatment of

A asthma
B infantile pyloric stenosis
C peptic ulcer
D diarrhoea
E heart block

19.11 In Parkinson's disease

A the basal ganglia are deficient in dopamine
B anticholinesterases improve movement
C reserpine replenishes dopamine stores
D chlorpromazine aggravates the condition
E amantadine improves movements by its anticholinergic effect

19.12 Levodopa

- A is a metabolic product of dopamine
- B penetrates poorly into the central nervous system
- C is not metabolized in peripheral tissues
- D causes nausea
- E causes cardiac arrhythmias

19.13 The following statements are correct:

- A Pyridoxine reduces the therapeutic effect of levodopa
- B Dangerous hypertension may occur if levodopa is taken with a monamine oxidase inhibitor
- C Reserpine antagonises the effect of levodopa
- D Tricylic antidepressants antagonise the effect of levodopa
- E Metabolites of dopamine interfere with tests for phaeochromocytoma

19.14 Bromocriptine

- A is a dopamine antagonist
- B has a longer plasma t½ than levodopa
- C can cause psychiatric disturbances
- D can cause livedo reticularis
- E is used to initiate lactation

19.15 In the treatment of Parkinson's disease

- A anticholinergic drugs are particularly effective in relieving hypokinesia
- B levodopa is particularly effective in reducing tremor
- C amantadine is as effective as levodopa
- D ankle oedema may be caused by amantadine
- E haloperidol improves hypokinesia

19.16 In the treatment of Parkinson's disease

A involuntary movements are an indication that too much levodopa is being taken

B postural hypotension due to levodopa may occur

C some benefit from levodopa can be expected in 80% of cases

D levodopa delays the progression of the underlying disease

E the 'on-off' phenomenon may be helped by increasing the frequency of dosing

19.17 The following statements are correct:

A Abrupt cessation of therapy for Parkinson's disease has no adverse consequences

B Benign familial tremor is alleviated by alcohol

C Propranolol may benefit benign familial tremor

D Acute dystonic reactions due to phenothiazines should be treated with i.v. levodopa

E Chorea is improved by drugs that reduce the effect of dopamine

19.18 The following statements about levodopa + dopa decarboxylase inhibitor combinations are correct:

A It is essential that the decarboxylase inhibitor should enter the central nervous system

B Combinations cause less nausea than does levodopa on its own

C When a decarboxylase inhibitor is added to levodopa, the concentration of levodopa in the brain can be maintained with only one quarter the dose

D Decarboxylase inhibitors interfere with active transport of levodopa by the small intestine

E Combinations are safe to use with monoamine oxidase inhibitors

20 Sympathomimetics, Asthma, Shock, Hypotension

20.1 Sympathomimetic substances which occur naturally in the body include

A isoprenaline
B dopamine
C noradrenaline
D adrenaline
E amphetamine

20.2 The following statements about the mechanism of action of sympathomimetic drugs are correct:

A Catecholamines act on post-synaptic adrenoceptors to increase formation of cyclic-AMP
B Theophylline inhibits the enzyme (phosphodiesterase) that destroys cyclic-AMP
C Theophylline potentiates the efficacy of adrenoceptor agonists on the heart, which is particularly hazardous when they are given together
D Theophylline potentiates the efficacy of adrenoceptor agonists on the bronchi which is therapeutically useful
E Adrenaline acts by releasing noradrenaline stored in nerve endings

20.3 The following statements about the effects of adrenaline and noradrenaline are correct:

A The classification of adrenoceptors is based on the observation that block of the whole range of actions of adrenaline could not be attained by a single drug
B There are two major classes of adrenoceptor

C α-adrenoceptor blocking drugs block the cardiac and vasodilator effects of adrenaline

D β-adrenoceptor blocking drugs block the vasoconstrictor effect of adrenaline and noradrenaline

E Relaxation of the smooth muscle of the bronchi and uterus is mediated by β-adrenoceptors

20.4 The following statements about the action of sympathomimetics are correct:

A Adrenaline has almost exclusively β-adrenoceptor agonist actions

B Noradrenaline has an approximately equal mix of α-and β-adrenoceptor agonist actions

C Isoprenaline has predominantly α-adrenoceptor agonist actions

D Amphetamine acts indirectly by causing release of noradrenaline stored in nerve endings

E Dopamine acts not only on specific dopamine receptors but also on α and β-adrenoceptors

20.5 The following statements about the action of sympathomimetics (i.v.) are correct:

A Noradrenaline infusion causes a rise of systolic and diastolic blood pressure with bradycardia

B Adrenaline infusion causes a rise of systolic and fall of diastolic blood pressure with tachycardia

C Isoprenaline or isoxsuprine cause little change in systolic and fall in diastolic blood pressure with tachycardia and uterine relaxation

D Dopamine causes cardiac stimulation with overall slight reduction in total peripheral resistance and increased renal blood flow

E Dobutamine has greater inotropic than chronotropic effects on the heart

20.6 **Hazards of overdose with sympathomimetic drugs include**

A consequences of intense vasoconstriction
B cardiac dysrhythmias
C heart block
D interaction with halothane
E fetal distress

20.7 **In the management of bronchial asthma with drugs**

A salbutamol is relatively selective for β_2-adrenoceptors, and tremor is an expected side-effect
B unwanted effects of salbutamol are more troublesome if it is taken by inhalation than if it is swallowed
C isoprenaline and orciprenaline are drugs of first choice because they are unselective between β_1 and β_2-adrenoceptors
D aminophylline acts as β-adrenoceptor agonist
E aminophylline is potentiated by severe cardio-pulmonary disease

20.8 **Clinically useful approaches to the relief of bronchial asthma include**

A inhalation of pollen just before the pollen season
B use of a β_2-adrenoceptor blocking drug
C use of a histamine H_1-receptor blocking drug
D use of a drug that reduces the response to antigen-antibody reaction
E use of a cholinergic drug

20.9 **Drugs which are useful in constant and intermittent bronchial asthma include**

A sodium cromoglycate
B salbutamol
C theophylline derivatives
D propranolol
E beclomethasone

20.10 Drugs which are useful in status asthmaticus include

A salbutamol
B sodium cromoglycate
C hydrocortisone
D aminophylline
E prednisolone

20.11 In status asthmaticus it is dangerous to use

A morphine
B a barbiturate
C an intravenous adrenocorticosteroid
D an α-adrenoceptor blocker
E a β-adrenoceptor blocker

20.12 Shock

A is a state in which there is anoxic tissue damage to vital organs
B may be caused by infections
C may be caused by loss of fluid from the circulation
D may be caused by cardiac damage
E is treated primarily by getting the blood pressure into the normal range with vasoconstrictor drugs

20.13 In a case of shock, when the patient's needs have been carefully defined, the following statements are correct:

A It may be useful to reduce peripheral vascular resistance by an α-adrenoceptor blocking drug
B It may be useful to increase peripheral vascular resistance by noradrenaline
C Dopamine provides a mix of adrenergic actions on heart and circulation that is least likely to do harm and may even do good
D If fluid has been lost from the circulation the absolute priority is to replace it
E Enormous doses of adrenocortical steroid should never be used

20.14 Angiotensin

A is formed in the body from monoamine oxidase
B causes vasoconstriction and so hypertension
C I is converted to the active angiotensin II by an enzyme which is inhibited by captopril
D is useful in shock to increase perfusion of the brain
E is useful in orthostatic hypotension

21 Hypotensive and Vasodilator Drugs, Adrenoceptor Blocking Drugs

21.1 Clinically useful hypotensive (antihypertensive) drugs may produce their effects by actions on

A arteriole resistance vessels
B venule capacitance vessels
C adrenal cortex
D central nervous system
E blood volume

21.2 Hypotensive drugs act on

A parasympathetic ganglia
B α-adrenoceptors
C β-adrenoceptors
D noradrenaline synthesis
E noradrenaline release

21.3 Hypotension with posture and with exercise is a particularly disadvantageous feature with drugs that act by causing

A diuretic effect
B synthesis of false transmitter
C adrenergic neurone block
D β-adrenoceptor block
E dilatation of capacitance vessels

21.4   **Glyceryl trinitrate**

A   relieves angina pectoris by dilating the venous and arteriolar systems

B   tablets should be swallowed whole because it is subject to extensive hepatic first pass metabolism

C   action lasts about 4 hours ~ 30 · *Action begins in 2*

D   should be given at once if myocardial infarction is suspected

E   induces tolerance which is a substantial disadvantage

21.5   **When glyceryl trinitrate tablets are prescribed for angina pectoris the patient should be told**

A   to take it to prevent pain

B   to take it at onset of pain

C   that if throbbing headache and palpitations occur he should take another tablet

D   that if he feels faint he should stand perfectly still and as relaxed as he can

E   to keep the tablets in a warm humid place e.g. a shelf over the bath

21.6   **Amyl nitrite**

A   is a non-volatile liquid

B   is provided in a glass capsule that breaks noisily

C   has a smell that attracts attention of bystanders

D   is a first choice drug for angina pectoris

E   is a true aphrodisiac

21.7   **Diazoxide**

A   is a thiazide

B   is a diuretic

C   is a vasodilator

D   is extensively bound to plasma protein

E   should be given intravenously very slowly because it binds to plasma protein so readily

21.8 Diazoxide

A is useful for long term control of hypertension
B causes sodium retention
C is particularly useful for hypertension during childbirth (labour)
D is useful in hypoglycaemia due to pancreatic β-islet cell tumours
E acts on arterioles (cardiac afterload) rather than on veins (cardiac preload)

21.9 Hydrallazine

A dilates veins rather than arterioles
B does not generally cause postural hypotension
C is particularly suitable for sole treatment of hypertension
D characteristically causes bradycardia
E is acetylated in the body and patients may be classed as slow and fast metabolizers

21.10 In heart failure, vasodilators

A can be useful in refractory cases
B relieve cardiac preload
C relieve cardiac afterload
D usefully reduce cardiac output
E that are used include organic nitrates and sodium nitroprusside

21.11 In obstructive peripheral vascular disease

A drug therapy is more likely to be beneficial in arteriosclerosis than in vascular spasm
B if the skin of the leg becomes warmer it can be assumed flow to the muscles is similarly improved
C nocturnal muscle cramps occur and may be relieved by quinine
D any benefit may be due to metabolic changes in the muscle rather than to vasodilatation
E on the whole, drug therapy is disappointing

21.12 **The following statements about α-adrenoceptor blocking drugs are correct:**

A They act by competition
B They cause peripheral vasodilatation
C They are liable to induce tachycardia
D They are first choice in managing angina pectoris
E Labetalol has both α- and β-adrenoceptor blocking actions

21.13 **β-adrenoceptor blocking drugs cause**

A reduction of heart rate
B increased myocardial contractility
C peripheral vasoconstriction
D bronchoconstriction
E reduced hepatic blood flow

21.14 **β-adrenoceptor blocking drugs**

A increase myocardial oxygen consumption
B may have agonist effect in addition to their antagonist effect
C may have a quinidine-like effect
D characteristically lower the blood pressure immediately on commencing therapy
E reduce maximal exercise capacity

21.15 **β-adrenoceptor blocking drugs are used in**

A hypertension
B anxiety
C hypothyrodism
D cardiac arrhythmias
E glaucoma

21.16 **Patients taking a β-adrenoceptor blocking drug may experience**

A exacerbation of existing heart block

B precipitation of heart failure where cardiac performance is dependent on sympathetic drive
C fatigue
D cold extremities
E hypoglycaemia if they are diabetic

21.17 The following statements about adrenergic neurone blocking drugs are correct:

A They diminish noradrenaline release from sympathetic nerve endings
B They diminish noradrenaline reuptake into sympathetic nerves
C Tricyclic antidepressants reverse their hypotensive effect
D Fenfluramine reverses their hypotensive effect
E A characteristic adverse effect is failure of male ejaculation without impotence

21.18 Methyldopa

A probably acts by causing the formation of a false sympathetic transmitter
B is relatively free from unwanted postural hypotension
C causes hyperactive behaviour
D causes haemolytic anaemia with positive Coombs test
E causes depression

21.19 Clonidine

A probably acts primarily on β-adrenoceptors in the brain
B acts on presynaptic α-adrenoceptors at the sympathetic nerve ending, activating the physiological negative feedback system that reduces noradrenaline release
C causes marked postural hypotension
D withdrawal, if sudden, may be followed by dangerous hypertension
E has a reputation for efficacy in menopausal flushing and migraine

21.20 Angina pectoris may benefit from:

A drugs which interfere with passage of calcium into cells: calcium antagonists

B vasodilators

C stopping smoking

D α-adrenoceptor block

E β-adrenoceptor block

21.21 Major physiological targets for drugs controlling high blood pressure include

A blood volume

B the thyroid gland

C the adrenal cortex

D cardiac output and contractility

E peripheral arteriolar resistance

21.22 In the control of hypertension

A where a single drug is used there is a tendency for homoeostatic adjustments to annul its effect

B drug combinations, where each drug acts at a different site, improve efficacy

C drug combinations, where each drug acts at a different site, reduce the incidence of unwanted effects

D even mild cases require a drug combination

E guanethidine and methyldopa are drugs of choice for mild cases

21.23 Where speedy control of blood pressure is needed

A propranolol is best

B labetalol is effective

C guanethidine is effective

D methyldopa is effective

E diazoxide is effective

21.24 Important aspects of monitoring drug-treated hypertensive patients include

A assuring patient compliance

B measuring plasma sodium concentration where a diuretic is used

C ensuring that sexual intercourse is infrequent or, better still, stopped altogether.

D knowing what self-medication the patient is taking

E encouraging the continuous use of appetite suppressant in cases of obesity

21.25 The following statements about phaeochromocytoma are correct:

A Hypertension is sustained, never intermittent

B In a hypertensive emergency a β-adrenoceptor blocking drug must be given first

C In a hypertensive emergency phentolamine is a drug of choice

D Preoperative treatment with both α- and β-adrenoceptor blocade should be given for several days

E An α-adrenoceptor blocking drug can be helpful in diagnosis

22 Digitalis (Cardiac Glycosides) and Drugs for Cardiac Dysrhythmias

22.1 Digitalis glycosides

A inhibit an ATPase responsible for sodium and potassium transport across cell membranes
B have a positive inotropic effect on cardiac muscle
C decrease myocardial excitability
D reduce vagal activity
E depress activity of cardiac conducting tissue

22.2 Digoxin given for cardiac failure

A should be continued indefinitely in all cases
B is especially valuable when the cause of failure is tamponade
C is generally more effective when the cause of failure is valvular disease rather than myocardial disease
D increases ventricular emptying
E shortens the duration of systole

22.3 Cardiac arrhythmia due to digitalis

A is more likely if a potassium-losing diuretic is used
B may be indicated by worsening cardiac failure
C is often indicated by a bigeminal pulse
D if in the form of multifocal ventricular ectopics can safely be ignored
E should not be treated by direct current shock

22.4 Digitalis glycosides

A shorten the PR interval on the ECG
B cause atrial tachycardia with atrio-ventricular block
C improve diastolic filling in atrial fibrillation with rapid ventricular response
D increase T wave amplitude on the ECG
E reduce the velocity of atrioventricular conduction partly through a vagal effect

22.5 The following statements about cardiac glycosides are correct:

A The t½ of digoxin is about 48 hours
B The t½ of digitoxin is about 170 hours
C Digoxin is eliminated mainly by the liver
D Digitoxin mainly passes unchanged into the urine
E In renal failure the distribution volume of digoxin is reduced

22.6 When administering digoxin

A the loading dose should be the same whether it is given intravenously or orally
B the subcutaneous route is preferred if the patient cannot swallow
C about one third of the loading dose, given daily, should normally suffice as the maintenance dose
D steady state plasma concentration can be expected within three days if a constant daily dose is given
E a steady state plasma digoxin concentration of 0.5 μg/L measured 6–9 hours after the last dose is an indication that the dose is too low

22.7   The following statements about digoxin are correct:

A   Patients with renal failure should receive normal loading doses but reduced maintenance doses

B   In general no adjustment of dose is needed for patients whose creatinine clearances exceed 60 ml/minute

C   Renal clearance declines with increasing age

D   Hypothyroid patients require reduced doses

E   Plasma concentration in excess of 1.7 μg/L are associated with increasing risk of toxicity

22.8   The following statements about cardiac glycosides are correct:

A   Bioavailability of digoxin tablets is 100%

B   Digitalis glycosides convert atrial flutter to fibrillation chiefly by the vagal effect of shortening the refractory period of atrial muscle

C   Medigoxin is less completely absorbed than digoxin

D   Ouabain acts on the heart within 5–10 minutes of an intravenous injection

E   Special caution is necessary if calcium is given intravenously to a digitalised patient

22.9   Adverse effects of digitalis glycosides

A   include altered colour vision

B   include gynaecomastia

C   are always accompanied by bradycardia

D   may necessitate intravenous infusion of potassium

E   may respond to phenytoin

22.10   Adverse effects of digitalis glycosides

A   due to oral overdose may be prevented by cholestyramine

B   if severe necessitate haemodialysis

C   may arise if quinidine is given to a digitalised patient

D   in the child only uncommonly include heart block

E   in the child commonly include vomiting and drowsiness

22.11 In the treatment of cardiac failure

A morphine gives relief partly by reducing preload
B in a patient with atrial fibrillation digoxin can safely be
   withdrawn once failure has cleared
C a low sodium diet is necessary in all cases
D aminophylline acts partly by venodilatation
E some antacids may jeopardize recovery

22.12 Cardiac cells of the

A conducting system are electrically negative (in the
   interior) in diastole
B sino-atrial node depolarise at the same rate as those in
   the atrio-ventricular node
C conducting system increase their rate of depolarisation in
   response to circulating catecholamines
D muscle type undergo spontaneous depolarisation – *does*
E muscle type relax when depolarisation occurs – *contract*

22.13 An antiarrhythmic drug

A of Class I has membrane stabilising activity
B of Class III interferes with the depolarising movement of
   Ca ions into the cell *4*
C of Class IV prolongs the effective refractory period and
   duration of action potential of cardiac cells *?*
D may have actions of two Classes
E of Class II may exert its effects by protecting the heart
   against adrenergically stimulated ectopic pacemakers

22.14 Quinidine

A prolongs the effective refractory period of cardiac cells
B prolongs the QT interval of the ECG
C is used to prevent ventricular tachycardia
D lowers plasma digoxin concentration
E causes diarrhoea

22.15 Procainamide

A has a membrane stabilising effect on cardiac cells
B prolongs the effective refractory period of cardiac cells
C has cholinergic effects
D is more likely to cause a systemic lupus-like syndrome in slow acetylators
E can cause hypotension

22.16 Disopyramide

A possesses membrane stabilising properties on cardiac cells
B prolongs the effective refractory period of cardiac cells
C has calcium blocking effects on cardiac cells
D has a positive inotropic action
E should be avoided in patients with glaucoma

22.17 Lignocaine

A has membrane stabilising properties
B reduces the effective refractory period of cardiac cells
C is not given orally because it is not absorbed from the gut
D if given as a constant intravenous infusion would reach a plateau concentration in the blood in 6–8 hours
E in standard doses achieves higher blood concentrations in patients with cardiac failure than in patients without cardiac failure

22.18 The following statements about cardiac antiarrhythmic drugs are correct:

A Mexiletine possesses membrane stabilising properties
B Mexiletine lengthens the effective refractory period of cardiac cells
C Phenytoin shortens the effective refractory period of cardiac cells
D Sotalol has membrane stabilising properties
E Sotalol lengthens the effective refractory period of cardiac cells

22.19 The following statements about cardiac antiarrhythmic drugs are correct:

A Practolol should not be used for the emergency treatment of cardiac arrhythmias because it causes the oculomucocutaneous syndrome
B Propranolol in overdose causes heart block
C Bretylium causes parotid pain
D Amiodarone shortens the effective refractory period of cardiac cells
E Amiodarone causes corneal deposits

22.20 The following statements about cardiac antiarrhythmic drugs are correct:

A Tocainide has a longer t½ than lignocaine
B Ajmaline resembles quinidine in its antiarrhythmic action
C The most important effect of verapamil on cardiac cells is interference with the depolarising sodium current
D Failure of response to antiarrhythmic drugs may be due to hypokalaemia
E Quinidine should normally be given by the intravenous in preference to the oral route

22.21 Stimulation of the vagus nerve

A causes tachycardia due to its effect on the sino-atrial node
B accelerates conduction in the bundle of His
C reduces the force of contraction of the heart
D shortens the refractory period of the myocardium
E decreases myocardial excitability

22.22 Clinically useful reflex stimulation of the vagus nerve may be produced by

A pressure on one eyeball
B pressing on both carotid sinuses simultaneously
C Valsalva's manoeuvre
D swallowing ice cream
E inviting the patient to put his fingers down his throat

22.23 Stimulation of the sympathetic nervous system causes

A tachycardia due to increased rate of discharge of the sinoatrial node

B increase in conductivity of the bundle of His

C decrease in force of cardiac contraction

D shortening of the refractory period of cardiac cells

E reduced automaticity of the heart

22.24 Paroxysmal atrial or nodal tachycardia

A may be terminated by vagal stimulation

B if accompanied by atrioventricular block should be treated with verapamil

C may be caused by digoxin

D may be due to thyrotoxicosis

E if recurrent may be prevented by a β-adrenoceptor blocker

22.25 Atrial flutter or fibrillation

A may be treated with digoxin by mouth if the need for therapy is not urgent

B which responds to direct current shock may be followed by arterial embolism

C is corrected more readily by direct current shock if the patient is taking digoxin

D if treated with quinidine alone may give rise to a dangerous increase in ventricular rate

E due to long-standing rheumatic valvular disease is suitable for attempted conversion to sinus rhythm

22.26 The following statements about cardiac arrhythmias are correct:

A Sinus bradycardia after myocardial infarction should always be treated

B Ventricular tachycardia frequently leads to ventricular fibrillation and circulatory arrest

C Ventricular premature beats may be regarded as benign if they occur near to the peak of the T wave of the ECG

D Atropine is of value in emergency treatment of heart block

E Some gaseous anaesthetic agents may interact with endogenous adrenaline to cause ventricular fibrillation

22.27 In cardiac arrest

A the organ most sensitive to hypoxia is the heart

B electrocardiographic evidence of asystole is mandatory before starting treatment

C the neck should be flexed fully to aid respiration

D the femoral or carotid pulses should be checked to assess the adequacy of external cardiac massage

E sodium bicarbonate is necessary to correct metabolic acidosis

23 Diuretics, Oedema, Urinary pH

23.1   Diuresis may result from

A   increase in cardiac output
B   correction of hypoproteinaemia by intravenous albumin
C   inhibition of antidiuretic hormone secretion
D   drug action on renal glomeruli
E   stimulation of renal tubular carbonic anhydrase

23.2   In the kidney diuretics act at the

A   proximal tubule by inhibiting active reabsorption of chloride
B   ascending limb of the loop of Henle by inhibiting active transport of water
C   cortical diluting segment by preventing sodium reabsorption
D   distal tubule by inhibiting the action of aldosterone
E   distal tubule by inhibiting the action of antidiuretic hormone

23.3   The principal renal site of action of

A   triamterene is in the ascending limb of the loop of Henle
B   spironolactone is in the descending limb of the loop of Henle
C   frusemide is in the proximal tubule
D   osmotic diuretics is in the distal tubule
E   thiazides is in the cortical diluting segment

23.4 **The following statements about the action of diuretics in the kidney are correct:**

A   Loop diuretics diminish the osmotic gradient between medulla and cortex

B   Diuretics which act on the loop of Henle have a lower maximal effect than do drugs which act on cortical tubules

C   Diuretics which act on the cortical diluting segment have steep dose-response curves

D   Diuretics which act on the distal tubule have a weak natriuretic effect

E   Thiazides usually remain effective even at glomerular filtration rates below 20 ml/min

23.5 **Potassium deficiency**

A   with thiazides is so common that all hypertensives treated with these drugs should receive potassium supplements

B   due to a diuretic is particularly likely to occur in patients on digoxin *if there is hyperaldosteronism, or is an carbenoxide*

C   is a complication of treatment with carbenoxolone *or mineralo-*

D   is revealed by increased amplitude of the T wave of the ECG *cortie*

E   may cause renal tubular damage

23.6 **Potassium replacement**

A   with potassium chloride is more effective than with other potassium salts because chloride loss occurs with high efficacy diuretics

B   using tablets may result in oesophageal ulceration

C   is better retained if it is not given at the same time as the diuretic

D   is essential when amiloride is used

E   with potassium chloride is best undertaken using enteric-coated tablets

23.7 Hyperkalaemia

A as a result of diuretic treatment is a special hazard in patients with renal failure

B causes muscular weakness

C increases if sodium bicarbonate is given

D can be corrected by infusion of dextrose and insulin

E causes myocardial effects which may be alleviated by intravenous calcium

23.8 Excessive use of diuretics may cause

A lethargy and sleepiness

B hypotension

C the blood urea concentration to rise

D dilutional hyponatraemia *Plasma Na get unusally (NB)*

E chronic saline depletion *but total sod↓*

23.9 The following statements about diuretics are correct:

A Amiloride causes hyperuricaemia

B Thiazides improve carbohydrate tolerance

C Loop diuretics reduce renal calcium loss

D Loop diuretics potentiate nephrotoxicity of cephalosporins

E Thiazides may prevent renal colic in patients with idiopathic hypercalcaemia

23.10 Thiazide diuretics

A can reduce urine volume in diabetes insipidus

B are more effective antihypertensive drugs than are the loop diuretics for equivalent natriuresis

C which are lipid soluble act for longer than those which are water soluble

D are uricosuric

E may cause thrombocytopenia

23.11 **The following statements about the loop diuretics are correct:**

A Frusemide has a steep dose-response curve
B Part of the effect of frusemide in relieving acute pulmonary oedema may be due to vasodilatation
C Ethacrynic acid may cause gastrointestinal bleeding
D The diuretic action of bumetanide lasts for 24 hours
E Ethacrynic acid taken by mouth may cause deafness

23.12 **The following statements about the potassium-sparing diuretics are correct:**

A Spironolactone abolishes the therapeutic effect of carbenoxolone on peptic ulcer
B Spironolactone may cause gynaecomastia
C Amiloride antagonises the action of aldosterone
D Triamterene antagonises the diuretic effect of thiazides
E Spironolactone is best used alone, without other diuretics

23.13 **The following statements about osmotic diuretics are correct:**

A They are only effective if they are completely reabsorbed in the renal tubule
B They reduce intracranial pressure primarily by inducing diuresis
C Intravenous sucrose can reduce intracranial pressure
D Pulmonary oedema may result from their use if renal function is impaired
E Urea can produce useful diuresis in patients with renal failure

23.14 **Carbonic anhydrase inhibitors**

A cause an alkaline urine to be formed
B cause a metabolic acidosis
C are more effective if used continuously, not intermittently
D may lead to the formation of renal calculi
E cause intraocular pressure to rise

23.15 The following statements are correct:

A The diuretic effect of dopamine is due to renal vasodilatation

B In high doses dopamine stimulates α-adrenoceptors

C Isosorbide is an osmotic diuretic which is well absorbed from the gut

D The cation-exchange resin, Resonium-A, is used to treat hypokalaemia

E Acetazolamide increases renal potassium excretion

23.16 When diuretic drugs are used

A their effectiveness can be gauged by monitoring body weight

B unpleasant restriction of salt in the diet is usually unnecessary

C overdose is suggested by rising blood urea concentration

D postural dizziness may result

E to treat hepatic ascites, preliminary paracentesis is desirable

23.17 Oedema

A may improve with bed rest

B may improve with correction of anaemia

C of acute renal failure should first be treated with an osmotic diuretic

D of hepatic origin should be treated with amiloride in preference to spironolactone

E may respond to frusemide intravenously when administration by the oral route has been unsuccessful

23.18 An alkaline urine

A encourages growth of E. coli

B increases the efficacy of sulphonamides

C increases renal elimination of amphetamine

D decreases the risk of crystalluria with sulphonamides

E reduces irritation in an inflamed urinary tract

23.19 An acid urine

A increases the antimicrobial efficacy of hexamine
B decreases renal elimination of salicylate
C prevents uric acid stone formation
D is produced by giving ascorbic acid
E is produced by administration of methionine

23.20 Ammonium chloride

A is partly converted by the liver into urea
B is used to test renal acidifying capacity
C is a potent diuretic
D is useful in the management of hepatic failure
E causes hyperchloraemic metabolic acidosis

24 Gastric Secretion, Drugs used in Peptic Ulcer, Purgatives, Constipation Diarrhoea

24.1 Gastric secretion

A of acid is increased in patients with gastric ulcer
B of acid is responsible for diarrhoea in the Zollinger-Ellinger syndrome
C is usually unaffected by anticholinergics
D tests usually involve the injection of pentagastrin
E of pepsin as well as of acid is increased by histamine

24.2 Antacids

A are given with the object of removing hydrogen ion
B consistently accelerate the rate of healing in gastric ulcer
C are more effective against pain if given frequently in small doses
D containing magnesium may produce alkalosis
E containing calcium are more likely to produce vomiting if taken with a lot of milk

24.3 Aluminium hydroxide

A relieves gastric pain quicker than sodium bicarbonate
B tends to produce diarrhoea
C is a less efficient antacid than magnesium carbonate
D may be of use in the management of renal failure since it binds phosphate in the gut
E should not be used in the presence of heart failure

24.4   Healing of a peptic ulcer

A   is promoted by propantheline only if it is given by injection

B   is not known to occur spontaneously

C   is not influenced by stopping smoking

D   is more likely to occur after treatment with carbenoxolone if the ulcer is gastric, not duodenal

E   is not accelerated by cimetidine, though pain is relieved

24.5   Carbenoxolone

A   alters the quality of gastric mucus

B   causes sodium retention

C   must be continued for six months once a course has begun

D   causes hypokalaemia which cannot usefully be antagonised by spironolactone

E   is more effective than gefarnate

24.6   Chenodeoxycholic acid

A   is a naturally occurring bile acid

B   inhibits cholesterol formation in the liver

C   when used to dissolve gallstones needs to be continued for 8 years

D   can be expected to dissolve calcified stones if they are small

E   should not be given to patients with chronic liver disease

24.7   Cholestyramine

A   is an ion exchange resin

B   binds bile acids in the bowel

C   increases jaundice if used in a case of primary biliary cirrhosis

D   should not be given at the same time as other oral drug therapy

E   relieves itching of obstructive jaundice after about two weeks

---

24.8 The following statements are correct:

A Metoclopramide hastens gastric emptying
B Charcoal is thought to aid the expulsion of gas from the intestine
C Carminatives relax the cardiac oesophageal sphincter
D Dimethicone is thought to help flatulence by lowering surface tension
E Products of seaweed are used to relieve symptoms of oesophagitis

24.9 Dietary fibre

A is not broken down by the enzymes of the gut
B intake of African rural people is more than twice that of urbanised Westerners
C accounts for less than 10% of the content of bran
D can be increased by eating wholemeal bread
E can reverse the anatomical changes of diverticular disease of the colon

24.10 Bulk purgatives include

A prunes
B magnesium sulphate
C dioctyl-sodium sulphosuccinate
D methylcellulose
E bisacodyl

24.11 Liquid paraffin

A has an unpleasant taste
B is best given as a suppository since only the last few feet of gut need lubricating
C if taken at night carries a risk of lipoid pneumonia
D is chemically inert
E carries a slightly increased risk of intestinal cancer if used continually as a laxative

24.12 **The following statements about stimulant purgatives are correct:**

A Rhubarb was originally used to 'denature' artificial wines
B Castor oil should never be taken on an empty stomach
C Cascara is obtained from an Arabian shrub
D Phenolphthalein turns alkaline urine red
E Neither aloes nor senna are available as biologically standardised preparations

24.13 **Purgatives**

A have a definite part to play in the treatment of obstruction of the bowel
B are essential to get rid of hardened masses of faeces in the rectum
C may be useful in hepatic coma
D should be avoided by patients taking broad spectrum antibiotics
E are not known to cause dependence

24.14 **In the treatment of diarrhoea**

A kaolin directly increases the viscosity of gut contents
B drugs of the opium group reduce peristalsis
C naloxone is ineffective against respiratory depression due to overdose of diphenoxylate
D anticholinergic drugs are valueless
E occurring in international travellers, codeine phosphate is likely to be more effective than antimicrobial drugs

24.15 **Treatment of a severe attack of ulcerative colitis includes**

A a broad spectrum antibiotic
B at least three litres of electrolyte fluid daily
C intravenous prednisolone
D hydrocortisone by intrarectal drip
E large doses of azathioprine

25 Histamine and Histamine H_1 and H_2-receptor Antagonists

25.1 Histamine

A occurs naturally in most tissues of the body
B acts as a local hormone
C is released from tissue stores in response to physical or chemical or immunological injury
D dilates the bronchi
E raises the blood pressure

25.2 Histamine

A decreases permeability of capillaries
B inhibits gastric secretion
C plays a role in urticaria and angioneurotic oedema
D has no role in seasonal hay fever
E produces effects all of which are blocked by all antihistamines

25.3 The following statements about histamine and antihistamines are correct:

A H_1-receptors occur particularly in the stomach and on vascular smooth muscle
B H_2-receptors occur particularly on the blood vessels
C Antihistamines are competitive antagonists to histamine
D In a life-threatening allergic reaction in which histamine release is a major factor (anaphylactic shock) the first line emergency treatment is a physiological antagonist, e.g. adrenaline, rather than a competitive histamine antagonist
E Antihistamines are remarkably selective and so free from other actions

25.4 Unwanted effects of histamine H$_1$-receptor antagonists include

A gastric ulceration
B central nervous system depression
C anticholinergic effects
D convulsions in overdose
E skin rash with topical application

25.5 Cimetidine

A is useful in gastric ulcer
B is useful in duodenal ulcer
C relieves pain of peptic ulcer without inducing healing
D used long-term delays relapse of duodenal ulcer
E is not effective in gastro-oesophageal reflux

26 Drugs and Blood Clotting, Blood-lipid Lowering Agents

26.1 In the blood coagulation system

A   damaged platelets are the only source of thromboplastin
B   thrombin catalyses its own production by liberating more thromboplastin from platelets
C   calcium ions are needed for the conversion of prothrombin to thrombin
D   plasma prothrombin concentration is low in newborn infants
E   fibrinogen contributes to the process of fibrinolysis

26.2 Vitamin K

A   is necessary for the formation of Christmas factor in the liver
B   requires bile for its absorption
C   restores reduced plasma prothrombin concentration to normal even in patients with considerable liver damage
D   is widely distributed in plants
E   deficiency may occur as a result of small intestine resection

26.3 When vitamin K is used

A   acetomenaphthone must be given intravenously since it is not absorbed from the intestine
B   phytomenadione (Konakion) is the most rapidly effective preparation
C   acetomenaphthone has a longer duration of action (several days) than menadiol sodium phosphate (Synkavit)

D a large dose may render a patient resistant to warfarin for about two weeks

E haemolysis may occur even with a low dose in a patient with glucose-6-phosphate dehydrogenase deficiency

26.4 Heparin

A was discovered by a medical student in the course of physiological research on blood clotting

B occurs in mast cells

C greatly enhances the activity of naturally occurring antithrombin III

D has a vasoconstrictor effect which limits its use in arterial embolism

E rarely requires the use of protamine sulphate to counter its effects

26.5 Treatment with intravenous heparin

A is required because the drug is precipitated by acid

B in a total daily dose of about 40 000 I.U. can be expected to ensure satisfactory anticoagulation

C by constant rate infusion pump is more effective than by repeated bolus

D can be effectively monitored only by measuring the thrombin time

E commonly induces mild thrombocytopaenia

26.6 Warfarin

A needs to be given in larger than usual doses to patients on antibiotics

B can be expected to achieve satisfactory control of coagulation in 7–10 days

C results in adverse allergic reactions about as often as phenindione does

D should on no account be stopped suddenly because of the risk of thromboembolism

E treatment only results in a serious risk of bleeding if the prothrombin time is prolonged above three times the normal value

26.7 The effect of anticoagulant treatment with warfarin is

A increased in patients taking aspirin
B increased in chronic alcoholics even where there is no evidence of liver damage
C reduced in patients taking oral contraceptives
D unaltered by tetracycline therapy
E not modified in diabetics by the use of oral hypoglycaemic agents

26.8 Anticoagulant treatment in established venous thromboembolism

A is more useful for a thrombus in a proximal large vein than one in a tibial vein
B should be continued for six months after a pulmonary embolus
C is contraindicated in the presence of pulmonary hypertension
D helps the recanalisation of veins
E is more useful than in a case of arterial thrombosis

26.9 Low-dose heparin administered subcutaneously

A has been clearly shown to reduce the incidence of postoperative thromboembolism
B may be more effective if combined with dihydroergotamine
C prevents pulmonary embolism in patients with established deep vein thrombosis
D produces troublesome spontaneous bleeding
E does not require laboratory monitoring

26.10 Situations in which oral anticoagulant treatment may be useful include

A   chronic atrial fibrillation
B   crescendo angina
C   a large myocardial infarct
D   prolonged immobilisation of a patient
E   symptomless hyperlipidaemia

26.11 Long-term anticoagulant therapy

A   if well conducted, carries no increased risk of haemorrhage
B   can be undertaken confidently provided that prothrombin estimations can be made every twelve weeks
C   provides no emotional problem for a patient without a long history of psychiatric disease
D   is best avoided in bacterial endocarditis
E   should in no circumstances be used in the presence of haemorrhoids

26.12 Oral anticoagulant treatment

A   may be teratogenic in early pregnancy
B   can cause haemorrhagic fetal death in the third trimester
C   precludes breast-feeding
D   provides particular hazards for patients undergoing prostatectomy
E   is best withdrawn five days before elective surgery

26.13 Bleeding in haemophilia can sometimes be stopped by

A   pressure
B   local application of an enzyme preparation from the venom of the Malayan pit viper (ancrod)
C   intravenous injection of human thrombin
D   topical fibrin foam
E   tranexamic acid after dental extraction

26.14 Streptokinase

A is best given by systemic infusion for the treatment of popliteal embolism
B is contraindicated for obstructed arteriovenous shunts
C activates plasminogen
D should not be given unless an antiplasmin such as aminocaproic acid is at hand
E should be used with caution in diabetic patients treated with phenformin

26.15 Altered platelet function

A occurs in Eskimos as a result of eating fat from cold-water animals
B follows imbalance between the formation of prostacyclin and thromboxane A_2
C does not follow treatment with clofibrate
D after aspirin treatment consists of modified aggregation and release reactions as well as altered stickiness
E may explain the beneficial effect of aspirin in patients with transient ischaemic attacks

26.16 Clofibrate

A has been shown in a large international study to reduce the incidence of fatal heart attacks in patients with high serum cholesterol concentration
B reduces plasma concentration of triglycerides to a greater extent than cholesterol
C interferes with oral anticoagulant control
D helps to prevent the formation of gallstones
E is more liable to produce adverse reactions in hypoproteinaemic patients

27 Pituitary and Sex Hormones, Contraception, Ergot, Prostaglandins

27.1   Genetic manipulation has resulted in the synthesis of

A   growth hormone
B   somatostatin
C   prolactin
D   pro-insulin
E   oxytocin

27.2   Somatostatin

A   causes vasodilatation
B   antagonises the effect of thyrotrophin-releasing hormone (TRH)
C   occurs in other parts of the brain as well as the hypothalamus
D   enhances the production of luteinising hormone (LH)
E   inhibits the secretion of gastric acid

27.3   Among the anterior pituitary hormones

A   somatotrophin derived from animals is ineffective in man
B   human chorionic gonadotrophin (HCG) has been superseded by a preparation from the serum of pregnant mares
C   prolactin is secreted only by women
D   corticotrophin has a plasma $t_{\frac{1}{2}}$ of about 15 minutes
E   gonadotrophins are of no value in the treatment of failure of spermatogenesis

27.4 Vasopressin

A increases water re-absorption in the distal renal tubule
B secretion is stimulated by nicotine
C deficiency may occur in hypopituitarism
D is a useful drug to raise the blood pressure
E should not be used to control bleeding from oesophageal varices if there is evidence of myocardial ischaemia

27.5 In diabetes insipidus

A thiazide diuretics sometimes have an antidiuretic effect
B glibenclamide may produce clinical improvement
C clofibrate is contra-indicated
D dilutional hyponatraemia may occur
E desmopressin is the treatment of choice

27.6 The syndrome of inappropriate antidiuretic hormone secretion (SIADH)

A is only caused by oat-cell lung cancer
B is subject to the normal homeostatic mechanisms
C may need treatment with infusion of hypertonic saline in acute cases
D may be usefully treated by demeclocycline
E is unaffected by chemotherapy to the causative tumour

27.7 Oxytocin

A is a drug which any doctor can use without danger
B has been used to discharge milk from engorged post-partum breasts
C obtained from posterior pituitary glands is safer than the synthetic product (Syntocinon)
D treatment mimics normal uterine activity
E administered by the buccal route is particularly likely to cause uterine rupture

27.8 Testosterone

A is necessary for normal spermatogenesis as well as for growth of the sexual apparatus

B is antagonised by clomiphene

C is of little value in the treatment of sterility due to testicular failure

D may be beneficial in fibrocystic disease of the breast

E slows the rate of closure of the epiphyses of bone

27.9 In treatment with androgens

A testosterone enanthate is given by intramuscular injection

B fluoxymesterone carries no risk of virilisation in the female

C methyltestosterone is the preparation of choice for the control of itching in hepatic cirrhosis

D adverse effects include salt and water retention

E norethandrolone is preferable to testosterone in osteoporosis

27.10 Cyproterone

A has an affinity for androgen receptors both on the hypothalamus and on target organs

B is a derivative of progesterone

C directly blocks the synthesis of testosterone in the testis

D is used in female hirsutism

E exacerbates acne

27.11 In the prevention of postmenopausal osteoporosis

A oestrogen treatment suppresses parathormone secretion

B calcium is virtually valueless

C methandienone (Dianabol) is as effective as oestradiol

D oestrogen treatment carries a risk of endometrial carcinoma which may be reduced by giving a progestogen concurrently

E tamoxifen is sometimes useful

27.12 When an oestrogen is prescribed

A. the dose for replacement therapy is not greatly different from that required to suppress lactation

B oestrone sulphate is thought to have fewer adverse effects than stilboestrol

C synthetic or semi-synthetic oestrogens (e.g. ethinyloestradiol) are much cheaper than oestrogens obtained from natural sources (e.g. oestrone)

D if a patient is intolerant of one preparation it is unlikely that another preparation will prove more acceptable

E nausea and vomiting may be troublesome

27.13 In oestrogen relacement therapy

A lifelong treatment leads to an increased incidence of myocardial infarction

B continuous treatment is preferable to interrupted courses

C the minimal effective dose should be given

D sequential treatment with a progestogen is unnecessary in a hysterectomised woman

E the required dose is about ten times greater than that used in high-dose contraceptive pills

27.14 Oestrogen treatment

A is indicated in large doses for prostatic carcinoma

B may control recurrent epistaxis

C may result in painful gynaecomastia in men

D may worsen diabetes

E inhibits lactation by the same mechanism that bromocriptine does

27.15 The following statements about progesterone or synthetic progestogens are correct:

A Preparations in the past have been discredited because doses were often inadequate

B Treatment is clearly beneficial in all cases of habitual abortion even if occurrence of true progesterone deficiency cannot be established

C Administration of a synthetic progestogen to the mother can virilise a female fetus

D A slow release progestogen formulation can be given via an intrauterine contraceptive device for local endometrial effect

E Danazol, derived from the progestogen ethisterone, is used for fibrocystic mastitis

27.16 In the control of conception

A testosterone inhibits spermatogenesis

B pheromones are likely to be useful in the near future

C vaginal preparations of ricinoleic acid are as reliable as copper-releasing intrauterine devices

D inactivation of pituitary gonadotrophins is best achieved by immunological techniques

E post-coital oral oestrogen treatment can only be effective within an hour of coitus

27.17 The effects of oral contraception with a mixture of oestrogen and progestogen include

A decreased viscosity of cervical mucus

B a substantial risk of harming an undiagnosed pregnancy

C decreased glucose tolerance

D liability to migraine

E an increased risk of developing rheumatoid arthritis

27.18 Users of oral contraceptives in Britain

A have a higher death rate than those using an intrauterine device in all age groups

B are more likely to develop cardiovascular complications if they smoke

C have a chance of about 1 in 3000 of becoming pregnant

D are not at increased risk for the development of gallbladder disease

E have more ectopic gestations than do vaginal diaphragm users

27.19 In the treatment of menstrual disorders

A the premenstrual tension syndrome is now generally agreed to be well controlled by bromocriptine
B dysmenorrhoea is usefully treated by inhibitors of prostaglandin synthesis
C menstruation can be advanced by giving norethisterone
D menorrhagia may be reduced by aminocaproic acid
E all cases of amenorrhoea should be treated by cyclical replacement therapy

27.20 The following statements about ergot derivatives are correct:

A Ergometrine and oxytocin have identical actions on the uterus
B Bromocriptine was produced for its prolactin-inhibiting effect
C Methysergide is a less active serotonin antagonist than is methylergometrine
D Co-dergocrine (Hydergine) can have modest beneficial effect on impaired mental function in the aged
E Postural hypotension is a recognised adverse effect of some

27.21 Prostaglandins

A are anti-inflammatory agents
B occur only in the seminal vesicles and central nervous system
C may cause uterine contraction or relaxation according to circumstances ·
D cannot yet be synthesised
E are formed from the same precursors as are thromboxanes and prostacyclins

28 Thyroid Hormones and Antithyroid Drugs

28.1 Thyroid hormone

A consists of T_4 and T_3

B exerts its effect chiefly through T_3, to which T_4 is converted

C is extensively bound to plasma proteins

D acts on specific receptors on target organ cells

E is stored in the thyroid gland as thyroglobulin

28.2 In the assessment of pituitary-thyroid function

A thyrotrophin-releasing hormone (TRH) estimation is an integral part of the T_3 suppression test

B radio-iodine uptake is reduced by large doses of salicylates

C TSH (thyrotrophin) can be measured in the blood

D investigation is made easier in patients already taking thyroid hormone by the negative feedback control mechanism

E particular difficulty occurs in some emotionally immature patients who are secretly 'addicted' to thyroxine

28.3 Treatment with thyroxine

A can reduce the size of puberty goitre

B for hypothyroidism in an old patient should start at a dosage of 1 mg daily

C need only be continued in a cretin until the age of five years

D is of great value in the routine management of simple obesity

E in an adult is difficult because the dosage needs to be changed so frequently

28.4 Liothyronine (T₃)

A finds its main use in myxoedema coma
B should not be given in a dose greater than 50 µg in 24 hours
C is best used mixed with thyroxine in tablets
D may cause heart failure if too vigorously used
E is more likely to cause exophthalmos than lid retraction

28.5 Iodine or iodide

A is present in most radiographic contrast media
B is an effective antiseptic
C ingestion, if continued, reduces the production of thyroid hormone transiently
D in very small amounts are useful in cough medicines
E may cause excessive salivation in intolerant patients

28.6 In the history of development of thiourea derivatives

A a team researching in the field of aplastic anaemia found that thiourea caused goitre
B the association of endemic goitre and hypothyroidism was only recognised after sulphathiazole was commercially produced
C phenlythiourea, as well as having a bitter taste, was found to cause goitre in rats
D research workers found that the goitrogenic factor in rape-seed was probably allylthiourea
E thiourea itself was used in the treatment of leprosy at the end of the nineteenth century

28.7 When drug therapy is used to control thyroid function

A perchlorate is most useful pre-operatively
B intravenous propranolol may be life-saving in a thyroid crisis
C β-adrenoceptor blockade is especially useful in thyrotoxic heart failure
D guanethidine eyedrops may improve lid retraction

E treatment should not be stopped whilst a thyroid bruit persists

28.8 **The following statements about the use of radio-iodine are correct:**

A All hyperthyroid patients treated with radio-iodine are likely to need treatment for hypothyroidism sooner or later

B A second dose should never be given

C Patients of child-bearing age should be advised not to get pregnant for a few months after treatment

D It has been shown that there is no increased risk of leukaemia even after the high doses required for treatment of thyroid carcinoma

E Radio-iodine treatment is preferable to surgery if there is obstruction of neck veins

29 Insulin, Oral Hypoglycaemics, Diabetes Mellitus

29.1 Insulin

A was discovered in Canada
B output by the pancreas is 30-40 units daily
C was easily standardised within a year of its first clinical use
D is stored in the liver
E is a polypeptide

29.2 Insulin causes

A reduction of hepatic output of glucose
B reduction of protein synthesis
C enhanced transit of potassium into cells
D stimulation of appetite, though its use for this purpose is obsolete
E reduction in the number of insulin receptors when the secretion rate is high, a factor in the insulin resistance of obese diabetics

29.3 When insulin is injected

A about half the dose can be recovered form the urine
B its plasma $t_{\frac{1}{2}}$ is about ten minutes
C and hypoglycaemia results, corticotrophin is released from the pituitary
D the intravenous route is preferred in severe ketoacidosis
E nowadays fat atrophy is unknown

29.4 The following statements about insulin preparations are correct:

A Insulin Zinc Suspension acts longer in its amorphous form than in its crystalline form

B Some allergic reactions occur as a result of proinsulin impurity

C New diabetics requiring insulin should ideally be started on HP (highly purified) or MC (monocomponent) insulin

D Soluble insulin should not be mixed in the syringe with Insulin Zinc Suspensions

E In North America insulin is only available in one strength

29.5 Soluble insulin

A is more likely to cause local discomfort if given at pH 3 than at pH 7

B if infused in a saline drip is subject to loss as a result of binding to the tubing

C has a peak action at 30-60 minutes when given intravenously

D is particularly useful for balancing patients who have heavy glycosuria before breakfast

E is the only preparation suitable for intravenous use

29.6 A hypoglycaemic attack

A should always be treated by sugar or glucose in the first instance

B which does not respond to glucose within thirty minutes suggests that dexamethasone may be useful as the patient may have cerebral oedema

C is never fatal

D should only be treated by glucagon injections if there has been no response one hour after intravenous glucose

E is less likely to occur in patients treated with insulin than in those on suphonylureas

29.7 The following statements about oral hypoglycaemic drugs are correct:

A Biguanides are effective even in the absence of insulin
B Sulphonylureas act by stimulating the β-islet cells of the pancreas
C Chlorpropamide is safer than tolbutamide in patients with poor renal function
D Lactic acidosis limits the use of biguanides
E Glibenclamide has the disadvantage of needing to be taken three times a day

29.8 In the treatment of diabetes it is generally accepted that

A patients should reduce their insulin dosage if they develop fever
B some drugs may interfere with both blood and urine glucose estimations
C it is best to control maturity onset diabetes by weight reduction alone
D once a patient has been stabilised on an oral hypoglycaemic agent, close supervision is no longer necessary
E good control of blood sugar reduces the incidence of neuropathy

29.9 In a pregnant diabetic patient

A oral hypoglycaemic agents are preferable to insulin
B insulin requirements fall during lactation
C the renal threshold for glucose rises in the third trimester
D maternal hyperglycaemia leads to fetal islet cell hyperplasia
E all treatment should be stopped during labour

29.10 Factors which can disturb the control of a diabetic patient include

A renal complications
B heavy dosage with sulphonamides

C large doses of aspirin
D the use of thiazide diuretics
E the use of oral contraceptives

29.11 In diabetic ketoacidosis

A it is sometimes difficult to decide whether to use insulin or an oral hypoglycaemic agent

B hypomagnesaemia is a problem as often as hypokalaemia

C insulin is best given by continuous low-dose infusion

D correction of acidosis by giving bicarbonate should take precedence over restoration of plasma potassium

E stringent precautions against septicaemia are necessary

29.12 In a diabetic patient undergoing major surgery

A a high blood glucose concentration, even for short periods, is particularly dangerous

B insulin is indicated even if there has been previous good control by oral hypoglycaemic drugs

C insulin requirements are likely to be higher as a result of operation

D glucose by mouth should be given one hour preoperatively

E ketoacidosis should be controlled, if possible, in all cases before operation, even in a surgical emergency

30 Iron, Vitamin B$_{12}$ (Cobalamin), Folic Acid

30.1 Iron

A stores are as easily replenished by oral therapy as by injection

B in haemoglobin accounts for less than ⅓ of total body iron

C released from destroyed erythrocytes is mostly excreted in the urine

D intake in the diet of an average Western man is 10-15 mg a day

E requirements in pregnancy are increased by over 2 mg daily

30.2 Absorption of iron

A is greater in an anaemic man than in a normal man

B is enhanced by ascorbic acid

C is easier if it is in ferric form

D is often reduced after partial gastrectomy

E takes place mostly in the upper small intestine

30.3 In iron deficiency

A transferrin provides a good measure of total iron binding capacity

B a high plasma ferritin is to be expected

C sore tongue is due to a reduction of iron-containing enzymes

D 25 mg of ferrous sulphate daily by mouth will produce a rise of 1% of haemoglobin per day

E it is important to give an initial loading dose of whatever iron preparation is used

30.4 In iron therapy

A iron dextran can only be given by intravenous infusion
B gastrointestinal upsets can be greatly influenced by the patient's anticipation of adverse effects
C tests for occult blood in the faeces are not generally interfered with
D intramuscular iron sorbitol causes the urine to turn black
E previously undetected folic acid deficiency is sometimes unmasked in the course of treatment

30.5 In acute iron poisoning

A symptoms are steadily progressive during the first 24 hours
B convulsions are to be expected within ½ hour of ingestion
C cardiovascular collapse is a feature
D an emetic is contraindicated
E raw egg and milk will help to bind iron until medical help is available

30.6 Desferrioxamine

A is excreted in the urine giving it a reddish colour
B in acute iron overdose should be given either orally or intramuscularly, never both
C can cause goitre by binding cobalt in the gut
D is indicated in some haemolytic anaemias as well as in haemochromatosis
E is available as an eye ointment for ocular siderosis

30.7 Vitamin B_{12}

A is now made from cultures of streptomyces
B can be absorbed independently of intrinsic factor if given in sufficiently large doses by mouth
C can be assayed microbiologically using Lactobacillus casei
D deficiency leads to intestinal malabsorption
E acts in megaloblastosis without any known effect on folate metabolism

30.8 Vitamin B₁₂ deficiency

A does not produce mental symptoms unless anaemia is present

B may occur following short term use of oral antibiotics

C occurring in jejunal diverticular disease can be remedied by tetracycline

D is best treated by hydroxocobalamin which is bound to protein to a greater extent than cyanocobalamin

E is often accompanied by hypokalaemia if it is vigorously treated

30.9 Folic acid

A alone provides adequate treatment for some cases of pernicious anaemia

B is absorbed in the large intestine

C is only active when converted to tetrahydrofolic acid

D is not present in green vegetables other than spinach

E should be used routinely in pregnancy in a dose of about 300 μg a day

31 Vitamins, Calcium, Bone

31.1 Vitamin A deficiency

A is to be expected in strict vegetarians
B leads to poor functioning of the rods of the retina
C occurs as a result of too much sunbathing
D should be thought of in a case of steatorrhoea
E causes epithelial damage

31.2 The B group of vitamins

A are all soluble in water
B includes pantothenic acid
C are found in large quantities in yeast and liver
D are not synthesised in any way in the body
E may become deficient in thyrotoxicosis

31.3 Thiamine deficiency

A is not usually accompanied by other vitamin deficiency
B should be considered in any case of obscure peripheral neuropathy
C may result in high output cardiac failure
D is likely to occur in populations who eat a staple diet of brown rice
E is confirmed if blood pyruvate falls after glucose has been given by mouth

31.4   The following statements about B vitamins are correct:

A   Riboflavine deficiency causes vascularisation of the cornea

B   Dementia occurs as a result of nicotinamide deficiency

C   Pellagra is less likely to occur in an underfed population if maize is the staple food

D   Pyridoxine can block the therapeutic effect of levodopa in Parkinsonism

E   Nicotinamide derived from tryptophan may be of use in the treatment of homocystinuria

31.5   Serious vitamin C deficiency

A   can be prevented equally effectively by all citrus fruits

B   causes bleeding gums in old people especially if they are edentulous

C   manifested as scurvy does not occur in any animal other than man

D   results in delayed wound healing

E   is more likely to occur in babies fed on cows' milk than on breast milk

31.6   Methaemoglobinaemia

A   impairs the oxygen carrying capacity of the blood

B   may be due to treatment with sulphonamides

C   is better treated in urgent cases with ascorbic acid than by methylene blue

D   can occur in a congenital form

E   responds less well to ascorbic acid than does sulphaemoglobinaemia

31.7   In tetany

A   hysterical overbreathing is a common cause

B   aluminium hydroxide by mouth may make things worse in patients with pyloric stenosis

C   a feeling or warmth spreading over the body after intravenous calcium has been given is a sign of danger

D cholecalciferol acts more quickly than dihydrotachysterol
E the use of parathormone is limited by the development of immunological resistance

31.8 In hypercalcaemia

A the heart is more severely affected in digitalised patients
B cardiac arrest is more likely to occur in cases of acute renal failure
C due to sarcoidosis calcitonin is more useful for long-term treatment than is prednisolone
D due to cancer may respond to mithramycin
E diuretics have no therapeutic role

31.9 The following statements about vitamin D are correct:

A Alfacalcidol is superior to cholecalciferol because it does not require renal hydroxylation to become active
B In primary, diet-deficiency rickets the therapeutic dose of vitamin D is 3000 to 4000 I.U. per day
C Calcium with Vitamin D Tablets BNF contain approximately the same amount of vitamin D as Calciferol Tablets Strong BP
D A large single dose of vitamin D has biological effects for as long as six months
E Epileptics on long term anticonvulsant therapy are prone to vitamin D deficiency

31.10 The pain of Paget's disease of bone may be relieved by

A improving the blood supply with tocopherols
B inhibiting bone resorption with calcitonin
C inhibiting crystal formation with diphosphonate
D inhibiting osteoclasts with a cytotoxic agent
E increasing osteocyte activity with parathormone

32 The Chemotherapy of Malignant Disease or Cytotoxic Chemotherapy, Immunosuppressives, Immunostimulants

32.1 In the chemotherapy of malignant disease the following statements are historically correct:

A The first attempt to control cancer by means other than surgery was not made until the end of the nineteenth century

B Observation that oophorectomy prolonged lactation in cows led to the suggestion that some cases of breast cancer are dependent on ovarian function

C The unreliability of plasma acid phosphatase concentration as a marker of activity held up the development of oestrogen treatment for prostatic cancer for several years

D Depression of haemopoiesis by sulphur mustards (the precursors of nitrogen mustards) was observed when they were used as chemical weapons in the 1914-18 war

E Nitrogen mustards had to be tested first on man since no satisfactory animal model was available

32.3 Success of chemotherapy in malignant disease depends on

A a good immune response to treatment

B the size of the tumour

C the number of cells dividing at any one time

D the endocrine environment of the malignant cell

E the rate of recovery of normal tissues from the effects of treatment

32.3 Cancer cells

A have less differentiated morphology than the tissue of origin

B divide more rapidly than the cells in any normal organ

C have a longer survival time if a large number are initially present

D are generally most sensitive to drugs when they are in a resting phase

E are not subject to the normal feedback mechanism which restricts cell multiplication

32.4 Factors which tend to make an ageing cancer less susceptible to drugs include

A increased capacity for metastasis

B increased cell cycle (division) time

C failure of normal marrow to recover quickly from the effect of cytotoxic agents

D exponential shortening of volume-doubling time

E overcrowding of cells, denying access to drugs

32.5 The following statements on principles of chemotherapy in cancer are correct:

A A given dose of drug kills a constant number of cells, however many are present

B Selectivity of drugs for cancer cells is less in lymphoma than in other tumours

C Some drugs only kill cancer cells in a particular phase of their active cycle

D Inadequate initial therapy is the usual reason for failure to control choriocarcinoma

E Resistance to drugs occurs as a result of factors which are quite dissimilar from those involved in the development of bacterial resistance

32.6 In planning intermittent combination therapy

A vincristine is used to synchronise active cell cycles

B most regimens have been devised on a basis of commonsense empiricism

C intervals between courses of drugs should be at least two months

D total cell kill is the object of POMP (prednisolone, vincristine, methotrexate and mercaptopurine) in acute lymphoblastic leukaemia

E overlap of toxicities between the drugs chosen is of little importance

32.7 Adverse effects of anticancer drugs include

A depression of both antibody and cell mediated immunity

B irreversible alopecia

C opportunistic infection with a protozoon (e.g. pneumocystis)

D urate nephropathy

E a temporary mutagenic effect on gonadal cells

32.8 In hormone-dependent cancer

A adrenocortical hormones, though useful for complications, have no direct action on the cancer itself

B prostate cancer is androgen-dependent

C breast cancer is less likely to respond to oophorectomy in post-menopausal than in premenopausal women

D a better therapeutic result in breast cancer can be attained in tumours having both oestrogen and progesterone receptors

E tamoxifen confers no benefit on post-menopausal women with breast cancer

32.9 In the immunotherapy of cancer

A tumour specific antigens have been found on a wide range of human tumours

B the place of BCG is dubious

C   immunisation with allogeneic tumour cells has only been shown to be of benefit in melanoma

D   the use of levamisole may be limited by granulocytopenia

E   attempts to stimulate immunity should not be made in the absence of a 'biochemical marker' such as α-fetoprotein

32.10   The following statements about cytotoxic agents are correct:

A   Alkylating agents interfere with normal DNA synthesis

B   Methotrexate competitively inhibits dihydrofolate reductase

C   Folinic acid (Calcium Leucovorin) terminates the action of methotrexate

D   Fluorouracil is a purine antagonist

E   Azathioprine is a pyrimidine antagonist

32.11   In the field of cytotoxic agents

A   radiophosphorus is the treatment of choice for polycythaemia vera

B   asparaginase is obtained from cultures of E. coli

C   vincristine causes cell cycle arrest

D   antibiotics such as bleomycin interfere with DNA/RNA synthesis

E   it is now generally agreed that Laetrile can relieve pain and prolong survival

32.12   Tumours in which significant benefit is common and life expectancy may become normal after chemotherapy include

A   multiple myeloma

B   oropharyngeal carcinoma

C   seminoma

D   squamous bronchial carcinoma

E   Wilm's tumour

32.13 One of the first choice drugs for

A chronic granulocytic leukaemia is busulphan
B Hodgkin's lymphoma is cyclophosphamide
C brain cancer is procarbazine
D ovary cancer is doxorubicin
E choriocarcinoma is actinomycin D

32.14 In immunosuppressive treatment

A established immunity is suppressed more readily than the development of an immune response after antigenic challenge
B cyclosporin A selectively inhibits multiplication of the immunocompetent T-lymphocyte
C response to a non-living poliomyelitis vaccine is diminished
D an early and vigorous approach is required in rheumatoid arthritis
E antilymphocytic globulin does not induce allergy

33 Drugs Acting on the Skin

33.1 When a drug is applied to the skin

A absorption is greater if an occlusive dressing is used

B healing of untreated distant lesions may occur

C it is of little importance what vehicle is used

D the consequences vary with the state of the keratin layer

E it cannot enter the deeper layers of the skin through hair follicles

33.2 Lotions

A are contraindicated in acutely inflamed lesions

B are less useful if there is much exudation

C exert their soothing effect through the evaporation of water

D are less often used than are creams in the alleviation of pruritus

E can reduce body temperature dangerously in old people

33.3 The following statements about skin creams are correct:

A An emulsion such as Zinc Cream, BP mixes with serous discharges

B Water-in-oil emulsions are more easy to spread than ointments

C Barrier creams are almost always capable of preventing occupational dermatitis

D Silicone sprays are useful in the prevention and treatment of pressure sores

E Masking creams are mostly used to protect against sunburn

33.4 In the therapy of skin disease

A non-emulsifying preparations such as Paraffin Ointment, BP are particularly useful on hairy areas

B pastes are ointments containing insoluble powders

C Zinc Starch and Talc Dusting-powder is likely to increase friction between skin surfaces

D insect repellents such as dimethylphthalate remain effective even in the presence of profuse sweating

E keratolytics may damage normal skin as well as soften horny layers

33.5 An alcoholic solution of chlorhexidine

A disinfects the hands if rubbed on till dry

B is the most suitable preparation for the disinfection of stainless steel objects

C is the disinfectant of choice preoperatively if diathermy is to be used

D is essential as a preliminary to venepuncture

E provides the best treatment for impetigo

33.6 The following statements about antiseptics are correct:

A 100% alcohol penetrates microbes more effectively than 70% alcohol

B Hexachlorophane is toxic to the central nervous system if absorbed through the skin

C Povidine-iodine has no antibacterial action in the presence of blood or exudate

D Hydrogen peroxide has a useful mechanical action as well as being a weak antimicrobial

E Cetrimide is a cationic surfactant

33.7 In the treatment of skin infections

A tetracycline combined with adrenal steroid is commonly used in children with infected eczema

B tinea responds to topical application of Benzoic Acid Compound Ointment, BNF

C if nystatin is used for candidiasis, it must be given systemically

D an allergic reaction commonly occurs with the use of penicillin on the skin

E griseofulvin is particularly useful in ringworm of the finger nails and hair

33.8 **Itching, when its cause is unkown or unremovable, may be alleviated by**

A Methyl Salicylate Ointment, BNF

B prostaglandins

C phenol

D aspirin

E crotamiton

33.9 **When an adrenocorticosteroid preparation is used in skin disease**

A systemic treatment should only be given in a serious condition such as pemphigus

B lichen planus can usually be controlled by dexamethasone

C psoriasis demands a high potency preparation such as clobetasol

D contact dermatitis from its other ingredients is prevented by the steroid in Quinoderm HC

E striae and purpura may follow local application

33.10 **Photosensitivity**

A may be produced by oral contraceptives

B sometimes follows the local use of deodorants

C can result in the inhibition of DNA and RNA synthesis

D can be prevented by the regular use of dihydroxyacetone

E in porphyria is best controlled by oral chloroquine

33.11 Phenylbutazone may cause

A erythema multiforme
B erythema nodosum
C exfoliative dermatitis
D chronic urticaria
E hair loss

33.12 Dermal adverse reactions

A to systemically administered drugs are commonly
   erythematous
B due to local contact are nearly always urticarial
C are usually of the same kind in all patients who take the
   offending drug
D recur at the same site in fixed eruptions
E usually only occur after a drug has been taken for months

33.13 Psoriasis

A can be rationally treated with oestrogen-containing
   creams
B is associated with increased numbers of horn cells
   containing abnormal keratin
C of the scalp is often treated by tar preparations
D can sometimes be helped by psoralens
E is unresponsive to adrenal steroids

33.14 Acne vulgaris may be usefully treated by

A sulphur-containing ointments
B vitamin A derivatives such as tretinoin
C systemic tetracycline
D oestrogens
E topical benzoyl peroxide

33.15 Adrenal steroids have a place in the treatment of

A alopecia areata
B seborrhoeic dermatitis
C herpes simplex
D rosacea
E sycosis barbae

33.16 The following statements are correct:

A Nappy rash is treated by a detergent such as cetrimide
B Pediculosis may respond to topical malathion
C There is no effective treatment for scleroderma
D Warts often disappear spontaneously
E Chemical depilatories make hair fibres swell so that they can be wiped off

34 Poisoning, Poisons, Antidotes

34.1 **In self poisoning**

A   most cases represent an attempt to commit suicide

B   domestic gas is still used as often as drugs

C   there is a mortality rate of about 1% of acute hospital admissions

D   the arthritic elderly are most likely to do it by accident

E   the drugs most commonly used are benzodiazepines

34.2 **In acute poisoning**

A   a selective antagonist is available for about 50% of cases

B   naloxone antagonises morphine

C   gastric lavage should be carried out at home before the patient is sent to hospital

D   if it is decided to induce vomiting, saline solution is the safest medicine to give

E   therapeutic emesis is contraindicated when petroleum products have been taken

34.3 **In the treatment of acute poisoning**

A   by a central nervous system depressant it is more important to sustain circulation than to wake the patient up

B   gastric lavage should be used in all cases of less than 4 hours duration

C   a cuffed endotracheal tube is sometimes indicated

D   it is unlikely that more than 30% of the ingested drug will be recovered whatever measures are taken to empty the stomach

E a stomach tube should not be used on an unconscious patient

34.4 Activated charcoal

A is in general of less value than raw egg and milk
B adsorbs both paracetamol and its antidote, methionine
C is most useful if given within an hour of ingestion of the poison
D is as effective in iron poisoning as is desferrioxamine
E should not be combined with an osmotic purgative in paraquat poisoning

34.5 In acute poisoning

A forced alkaline diuresis can be expected to be particularly helpful in phenobarbitone poisoning
B it is an advantage for a drug to be highly protein-bound when haemodialysis is undertaken
C peritoneal dialysis is an adequate alternative to haemodialysis in salicylate poisoning
D digoxin is more easily dialysable than is aspirin
E haemoperfusion is more useful than dialysis for a lipid soluble drug such as methaqualone

34.6 In the care of a patient unconscious due to drug overdose

A analeptics are preferred to assisted respiration
B moving the patient every three hours will prevent bladder distension
C an antibiotic alone will prevent hypostatic pneumonia
D there is no special indication for taking the temperature regularly
E dehydration must be prevented by giving parenteral fluid with nothing by mouth

34.7 Dimercprol

A acts by binding metal ions to its -SH groups
B may be life-saving in arsenic poisoning
C is only useful in lead poisoning if combined with calciumedetate
D is given by deep i.m. injection which causes pain
E causes hypertension

34.8 The uses of edetates include treatment of

A lead poisoning by intravenous sodium calciumedetate
B hepatolenticular degeneration in combination with penicillamine
C hypercalcaemia by disodium edetate
D cyanide poisoning by cobalt edetate
E some cases of paraquat poisoning

34.9 D–penicillamine

A is more effective than dimercaprol in hepato-lenticular degeneration (Wilson's disease)
B has to be given by injection
C has some beneficial effect on collagen disease
D causes no important adverse reaction
E can be substituted by penamecillin if it is not tolerated well

34.10 In cyanide poisoning

A early symptoms are similar to those of anxiety
B emergency treatment includes inhalation of amyl nitrite
C chelating treatment is similar to that used in tetraethyl lead poisoning
D sodium thiosulphate is useful in the later stages of treatment to release cyanide from methaemoglobin which has been produced in response to emergency treatment
E treatment differs from that of carbon monoxide poisoning in that there is no place for hyperbaric oxygen

34.11 The following statements about herbicides and pesticides are correct:

A Dinitro-orthocresol is not absorbed through the skin

B It is dangerous to use atropine to control sweating in poisoning by dinitrobutylphenol

C All rodenticides cause convulsions

D Paraquat is selectively taken up in the lungs

E Fuller's earth or bentonite should be given urgently in paraquat poisoning

34.12 CS, a common anti-riot agent

A is a solid used in aerosol form

B causes persistent bronchospasm even in normal people

C induces a transient rise in intraocular pressure

D has a plasma t½ of about 5 seconds

E causes excessive salivation which may persist for an hour

34.13 Drugs which have probably been used for torture or 'interrogation' include

A cyclophosphamide

B amphetamine

C thiopentone

D suxamethonium

E apomorphine

Answers

Chapter 1

Question	Answer
1	BDE
2	ABCDE
3	BCD
4	CE
5	AD
6	ABCDE
7	BDE
8	CDE
9	BDE
10	BCE
11	BC
12	ADE
13	AB
14	ABCD
15	CDE
16	ACDE
17	C
18	AD
19	CDE
20	ABCDE
21	AE

Chapter 2

Question	Answer
1	ABD

Chapter 3

Question	Answer
1	BCDE
2	ABCE

Chapter 4

Question	Answer
1	ABE
2	CDE

Chapter 4 (contd)

Question	Answer
3	CDE
4	DE
5	AD
6	ABCDE

Chapter 5

Question	Answer
1	CD
2	C
3	ABCDE
4	ABD
5	ABCE
6	BCD
7	ACE
8	B
9	BE

Chapter 6

Question	Answer
1	ABCD
2	ABCDE
3	ABCDE
4	BDE

Chapter 7

Question	Answer
1	ABCD
2	ACD
3	ABE

Chapter 8

Question	Answer
1	ABCDE
2	AC
3	CDE
4	ABE

Chapter 8 (contd)

Question	Answer
5	AE
6	BC
7	ACD
8	ADE
9	BDE
10	CD
11	ACDE
12	AE
13	ACDE
14	ABDE
15	CDE
16	ACD
17	ABCDE
18	CE
19	ACDE
20	C
21	ACD
22	ACE
23	ABD
24	BCE
25	BDE
26	ADE
27	ABDE
28	ABCDE
29	ABCE
30	CD
31	ABCD
32	ABCDE
33	BC
34	ACD
35	ABCE
36	AC
37	ABCD
38	AC